GETTING to the ROOT

YOLANDA M. LENZY, MD, MPH

Disclaimer: This book is not intended as a substitute for the medical advice of a physician. The reader should regularly consult a physician in matters relating to his/her health and particularly with respect to any symptoms that may require diagnosis or medical attention.

DEDICATION

To all of my patients (past, present, and future),
I wrote this with you in mind. I pray that these
words help you to get to the ROOT.

To my family and the "cloud of witnesses"
who have gone before me (Hebrews 12:1, KJV),
I pray this work
and my journey make you proud.

ACKNOWLEDGEMENTS

Thank you to my circle of family and friends who have walked with me through the completion of this "labor of love." Words cannot express my appreciation for every minute spent proof-reading, providing feedback on the cover or simply providing me with an encouraging word. This "God-given assignment" is an important work and it will help many people.

To my parents, thank you for the "good ground" that you watered and planted me in. To my sister Lila, thank you for allowing me to share your story. I am certain that it will help many. To my spiritual mentor and friend Dr. Gayle Jones, you are the real MVP. You read every word of this work and provided timely feedback and I am so grateful to have you in my life. To Kim Rennis, Regina Tillery-Jenkins, Shakenna Williams, and Dayo White, thank you for all that you do to help me shine! You are appreciated. To my office staff, thank you for taking every call from those looking for this book and for your feedback on the cover. Thank you to Ayisha Hayes-Taylor and Stephanie Parrott for all of your help in getting my thoughts out of my head and onto paper. Thank you to my business coach Mia Redrick and your team for supporting me through the completion of this book with excellence!

To my mentors: Dr. Lynn McKinley-Grant, thank you for being the role model that piqued my interest in Dermatology when I was 13 years old and started me on this journey. To my cosmetology instructor Mrs. Melanie Stancliff, thank you for believing in my dream to become a licensed cosmetologist and board-certified dermatologist one day and for supporting my involvement in student leadership. To Dr. Barbara A. Gilchrest, thank you for being the true definition of a mentor. Your advocacy and granting me a "seat at the table", made this possible. To Dr. Lynne Goldberg, thank you for all that you taught me in the Hair Clinic at Boston Medical Center and for supporting my idea to start educating hair stylists on hair loss when I was a first-year resident over 10 years ago! To my dermatology colleagues, thank you for your support in referring patients, pre-ordering and telling your patients about this work. That means the world to me!

To every cosmetologist and trichologist that I have worked with, thank you for your support, and I pray that this book will support you in your work with your clients. To every patient, thank you for all that you have taught me; you helped me to become a better physician. To everyone who views, likes and shares my Lunch & Learn with Dr Yolanda episodes, I appreciate you!

To my good friend J.C., thank you for your support and helping me think through the name Kingdom Root Publishing. I can't wait for the other books and authors that will be birthed out of this effort.

With gratitude,

Yolanda M. Lenzy, MD, MPH

TABLE OF CONTENTS

FORWARD

What makes a doctor exceptional? CARING. In her opening chapter to this "Guide to Understanding Hair," Dr. Yolanda Lenzy describes wanting to help others from early childhood. With this accessible, highly informative book, Dr. Lenzy will achieve her goal for many people, particularly for women of color, whose special hair problems have previously received far too little attention.

I first met Dr. Lenzy as a newly minted physician pursuing a public health degree. Because she also wished to explore basic research as a possible career path, I was pleased to offer her a post-doctoral fellowship in my laboratory at Boston University (BU). Ultimately, Dr. Lenzy chose to return to clinical medicine and entered BU's dermatology residency program. After three years of intense training, she took a special interest in the under-studied problem of hair loss that affected many of her patients at our safety-net hospital. Recognizing her passion for the subject, I invited her, still a trainee, to co-author a major textbook chapter describing intrinsic hair differences and consequent clinical hair problems in black men and women.

Dr. Lenzy now directs a successful dermatology practice, providing high-quality care for all of her patients, but with a focus on treating ethnic hair loss,, an expertise that has mostly been unavailable. Throughout this book, Dr. Lenzy is sharing her knowledge and advice with a far larger group of people who suffer from hair loss, as well as with the hair stylists to whom they often turn for help. Even physicians, including many dermatologist colleagues, will find the Guide a valuable resource for patient care. I count myself among them.

Barbara A. Gilchrest, M.D.
Chair-Emeritus, Department of Dermatology
Boston University School of Medicine
Department of Dermatology
Massachusetts General Hospital
Boston, MA

WHY I WROTE THIS BOOK

Aiming to eliminate the sunlight out of my eyes, I stood up to close the window shade near my sister, Lila. We had been in the kitchen the better portion of the day laughing, talking, and cooking. Thanksgiving this year was held at my home and I was overjoyed to have my entire family spending the holiday with us. As I stood over my sister, I immediately noticed something I had not seen before. The crown of her scalp was thinning. Not wanting to alarm her, I calmly asked if she had noticed it. Shocked by my discovery, she spun around in her chair, simultaneously running her fingers through the crown of her head, and gasped, "No!" The fullness of the front, sides, and back of her hair had camouflaged the process taking place in her crown. As a dermatologist, I was not surprised by her response. I see many patients in my office everyday who have no idea that their crowns are thinning until much later, sometimes not until the thinning has formed a distinct bald spot.

After I took a picture of my sister's scalp on her phone and zoomed in to show her the hair follicles, I told her I suspected she was suffering from the #1 cause of hair loss in African American women called CCCA or Central Centrifugal Cicatricial Alopecia. She was somewhat familiar with the condition because our mother, grandmother, and several of our aunts had also been diagnosed with it. CCCA (see Chapter 10) is a form of scarring alopecia that results in permanent hair loss. The scarring typically starts in the crown or central scalp and spreads outward or "centrifugally" over time. The good news is that identification, education, and the proper treatments can slow down the progression of hair loss. I reassured my sister of this and referred her to one of my dermatology colleagues who has a practice in her area and started her on a regimen right away. As a loving little sister, I followed her progress and gave advice, solicited or not. Like many patients, despite me discussing the importance of staying consistent with the treatment regimen, she would often forget and within 9 months the condition had significantly progressed (Fig. 1A – 1C).

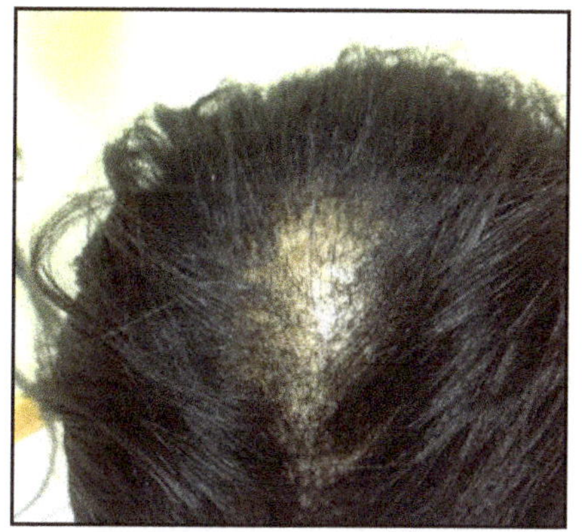

A) Pre-Treatment: Stage 2B

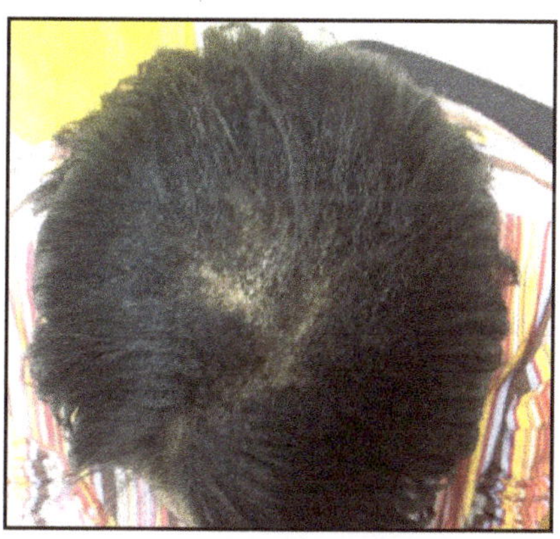

B) After 5 Months of Topical Steroids:
Improvement to Stage 1B

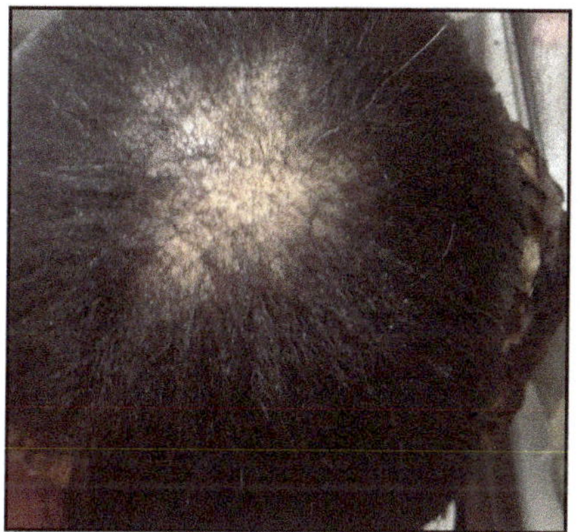

C) After 9 Months of Inconsistent Use of
Topical Steroids: Progression to Stage 3B

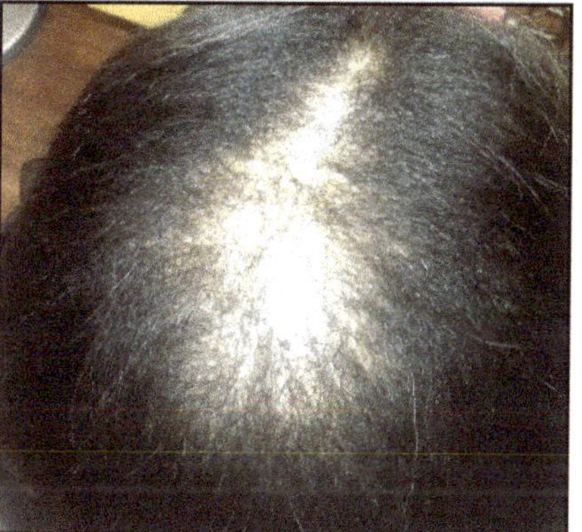

D) After 1 Year with No Treatment:
Progression to Stage 4B

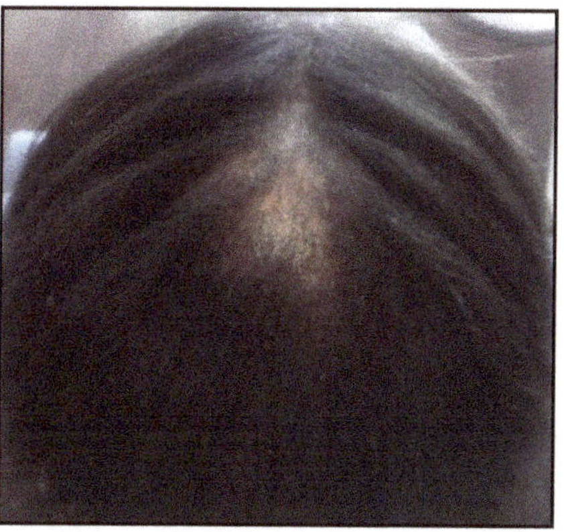

E) After 3 Monthly Steroid Injections:
Improvement Back to Stage 3B

As I often tell my patients, the treatments don't work sitting inside the tube or bottle. They must be used! I had to remind my sister of this as well. After the CCCA progression, I recommended a more aggressive treatment approach with steroid injections (see more about this in Chapter 10), which resulted in significant improvement (Fig. 1D and 1E). Since those early years, she has been committed to her treatment plan and faithful to following the recommended regimen. I like to believe the extra "encouragement" that she had from me has also helped her stay consistent over the past few years. Of course, she would probably refer to it more as "nagging" than "encouragement" but hey, that's what little sisters are for!

That is what I do every day. I ask the right questions, perform an examination, and make the diagnosis. But, making a diagnosis is only the first step. One of the vital functions that I serve as a dermatologist is to provide excellent patient education. The word "Doctor" is derived from the Latin verb *docere,* which means "to teach." In both my practice and virtual consultation service, while many of my patients have already seen their primary care physician (PCP), or another dermatologist, for the problem they are consulting me on and sometimes even had a biopsy performed, many patients still are unable to articulate their diagnosis. It could be that they just forgot or simply do not recall the details. This is the reason why I love providing my patients with written handouts or pamphlets so that I can ensure they have their actual diagnosis and a little more information about the condition, including the possible cause and treatment options. Or many patients state that the doctor went straight to the recommended treatment omitting in-depth details of the diagnosis. I like to counsel my patients on the WHO, WHAT, WHERE, and WHY (when it is known)—on how long their condition may last and exactly what they need to do, step-by-step. My sincere hope is that through this provision of health education, my patients feel empowered after their office visit. My passion and fulfillment comes from helping people overcome any hair or skin problem, helping them to achieve their hair and skin goals.

The practice of medicine is both an art and a science. The *science* is making the correct diagnosis and selecting the proper treatments, but the *art* of medicine is what I think distinguishes the "good" from the "great" professional and what distinguishes me as a dermatologist. My strength is explaining the complex scientific process behind a form of hair loss or a rash in ways that my patients can understand. I love to see what I call the "light bulb of understanding" come on with a head nod or raised eyebrows, which let me know that what I am explaining makes sense! Even more, I love to prescribe a treatment regimen and see the look of delight on my patients' faces at the follow-up visit when the advice and treatment that I provided actually helped them to get better and their condition to improve. This is what I love about what I do. As a dermatologist, I get to visually SEE the fruits of my labor. Whether it's arrested hair loss, pimples and/or dark spots vanished, or thicker, fuller hair, it's very rewarding to help patients in this way.

I am in a unique position as both a dermatologist and a licensed cosmetologist to help patients and clients deal with hair loss from a medical as well as an aesthetic perspective. My expertise is rooted in my extensive and unique training and experience. As a cosmetologist, I have the pleasure of using my training in product ingredient knowledge, hair cutting, coloring, and styling to help my clients undergo amazing transformations and achieve healthier hair. As a dermatologist, I have the opportunity to help that patient who is struggling with a problem by making a diagnosis and devising a plan to overcome or better manage the issue. This is what makes my practice unique. To my knowledge, I am the only dermatologist who is also a licensed cosmetologist. I have worked with patients who were suffering from hair loss and scalp disorders due to one of the 16 major types I will introduce to you in this book. I have included two additional chapters on natural hair and nutrition to complete our discussion:

1. Telogen Effluvium (Ch 2)
2. Androgenetic Alopecia (Ch 3)
3. Alopecia Areata (Ch 4)
4. Trichorrhexis Nodosa (Ch 5
5. Traction Alopecia (Ch 6)
6. Tinea Capitis (Ch 7)
7. Trichotillomania (Ch 8)
8. Anagen Effluvium (Ch 9)
9. CCCA (Ch 10)
10. LPP & FFA (Ch 11)
11. Dissecting Cellulitis of the Scalp (Ch 12)
12. Folliculitis Decalvans (Ch 13)
13. Acne Keloidalis Nuchae & PFB (Ch 14)
14. Discoid Lupus Erythematosus (Ch 15)
15. Seborrheic Dermatitis (Ch 16)
16. Psoriasis (Ch 17)
17. Going Natural (Ch 18)
18. Nutrition & Hair (Ch 19

In addition, my experience includes providing solutions for men and women who are suffering from life-threatening illnesses such as cancer (in all forms), which in turn, may result in hair loss as a secondary effect. In these cases, my work consists of much more than the aesthetic. The confidence and sense of normalcy that can be restored to those affected by life-threatening diseases by giving them the tools needed to combat/camouflage their hair loss is immeasurable for them and for me and truly embodies why I do this.

Education, clinical training, and scope of practice are critical in the treatment of hair loss. I have noticed on social media great confusion around the roles of the various professionals who can assist in the management of hair loss. I want to take a moment to define the various professionals and their scope of practice. On the great "YouTube University," I have seen it erroneously stated in videos that dermatologists solely specialize in the skin and trichologists are the experts of hair and scalp disorders. Dermatologists are the *physician experts* of any condition involving the hair, skin, and nails. Trichologists, on the other hand, are *para-professionals* (typically cosmetologists in the United States) who have received additional training in hair and scalp conditions. However, they are not licensed to practice medicine, make diagnoses and to provide the full gamut of available treatment options that a dermatologist is medically certified to offer. A well-trained trichologist can provide counseling and supplemental hair and scalp and over-the-counter nutritional treatments. It is important to note that trichologists lack the ability to perform biopsies, order diagnostic tests, and prescribe medications, which are often needed for many of the hair and scalp conditions that we will discuss in this book. I do work with many excellent trichologists as part of a client's "hair loss team," in which I provide the medical management and they provide the hair care management. It is very important that clients working with a trichologist work with a dermatologist as well to ensure the client has an accurate diagnosis and access to the full range of available treatments, prescriptions, and over-the-counter nutritional treatments.

Incorrect advice can delay critical intervention that could accurately address the issue. Unfortunately, I've seen many cases that could have been prevented if a patient had opted for early medical consultation and treatment verses self-diagnosis by way of the Internet. That is one of the reasons why I felt it was so important to write this book. While I frown upon self-diagnosis, I am a huge advocate of patients empowering themselves with credible information. Being able to qualify your symptoms and medical history, including time progression, so that you may speak from a place of familiarity with your physician when you are able to see one, could make all the difference in your confidence, as well as your clarity.

ARRIVING AT DERMATOLOGY

I did not always know I wanted to become a doctor, but I have always known I wanted to help people look and feel better about themselves. During middle school, I developed a passion for hairstyling. My dad styled my hair in elementary school because my mother went to work very early in the morning. As soon as I was old enough, I told him I wanted to do it myself and I guess I did a pretty good job because as my skills improved, my mother and my sister trusted me to do their hair as well. My family affirming those talents early on only convinced me even more that I was on a path that I wanted to continue. My mother even told other people outside of our immediate family that I gave the best scalp massages and everyone wanted me to shampoo their hair! It became a weekend ritual at our home. Shampooing naturally progressed to blow drying and styling, and just as anyone who wanted to hone their craft would do, I started studying the professionals. When I would go to the salon, I would watch every detail of the stylists' work. I was very observant. I picked up how to use a curling iron and blow dryer, and the intricate details that stylists practiced to create their art. From the brands of tools they used, to the flicks of their wrists while using them, I absorbed every detail like a sponge.

When it was time, I decided to pursue a non-traditional educational path of enrolling at Laurel High School. It was the only high school in our county that offered vocational training in cosmetology as well as a college preparatory track called the University High School. No prior student had enrolled in both programs simultaneously, but I didn't let that hinder me. In my freshman year, I met with the vice principals of both programs and informed them of my goals to obtain my license in cosmetology and then matriculate to college after graduation. I laid out a plan that I wanted to enroll in BOTH the vocational education and the college prep tracks with my core academic subjects in the college preparatory track. They told me that no one had ever done that before. My response was, "Can I be the first?!" They looked at my transcripts and saw that I was an excellent student and could not think of one good reason why I couldn't. Therefore, in 1991, I became the first student simultaneously admitted to the university and vocational tracks.

During my sophomore, junior, and senior years, I studied cosmetology for three hours a day; for the other part of the day, I took college preparatory English, Math, History, and Science. My cosmetology instructor, Mrs. Melanie Stancliff, observed my leadership skills and encouraged me to pursue my aspirations in the organization for students enrolled in vocational education called, the Vocational Industrial Clubs of America (now SkillsUSA). In my senior year, I was elected National Vice President for VICA, which was one of the best personal development experiences that I have experienced to date. By the end of high school, I had accumulated enough hours to sit for the state board cosmetology exam. I passed the exam and became a licensed stylist right out of high school. I was able to professionally do hair out of my dormitory room at American University as a way to support myself in college, outside of the full academic scholarship that I received.

As much as I enjoyed cosmetology, I wanted to pursue my second passion—to understand how to help my clients from a medical perspective. When I was 14 years old, my mother took me to see a dermatologist where she worked at the MedStar Washington Hospital Center because I had horrible eczema. The doctor's name was Lynn McKinley-Grant. Encountering Dr. McKinley-Grant changed my life. Not only was she a smart, beautiful, professional woman, she also looked like ME! This was my first time ever being cared for by an African American female physician and, needless to say, my interest in medicine was piqued. My mother worked at the same hospital delivering food to the patients, which is how she came to know about Dr. McKinley-Grant. After my initial doctor's appointment with her, every time my mom would see her around the hospital, she would tell Dr. McKinley-Grant, "My daughter is always saying how much she admires you!" This led to Dr. McKinley-Grant stopping to talk to my mom while she was doing her rounds and they would talk about me. Eventually, Dr. McKinley-Grant invited my mom to bring me in for a visit to shadow her in the office. This led to her becoming my mentor. I am so grateful to my mom for stepping forward and facilitating our relationship to blossom.

My mother loved the medical field, but had little opportunity for formal training. Growing up in Greenville, North Carolina, her family sharecropped a tobacco farm when she was young. She has described multiple instances when she couldn't attend school in September because the tobacco had to be harvested. That's how it was for many sharecropper families. During certain times of the year, school was secondary. However, my mother kept me focused on learning and never let her dream of a physician-daughter wane, constantly pushing and encouraging me, saying, "You can do it!" If I had lots of chores and homework to do, there were even some nights where my mom would take over my chores so that I could study, much to my dad's disapproval. Don't get me wrong, my dad wanted me to achieve my goals and dreams, too, but he was not about skipping out on those chores!

My mom just wanted me to focus and never doubted for one moment that education would give me wonderful options for my life. I think she wanted more for me and my sisters because of what she experienced at the hospital. She experienced painful varicose veins from standing on concrete floors and working on her feet all day in a freezer. She had a tough time preparing the patient trays in such extreme conditions, and would become uncomfortably cold. Despite all of those things, my mother worked faithfully to provide the best of care that is required to work in the health care industry. The hard things she faced every day caused her to push us to accomplish more because she could see how being a professional would give us many more opportunities than she had. Between my mother and father, I couldn't help but develop a stellar work ethic and a well-mapped education. I thank God for the work ethic that my father instilled in me because obtaining that education provided its own set of challenges.

Dermatology is an extremely competitive specialty to secure a position in a residency program. The Step 1 exam, which medical students take in their second year, is used as a factor in determining a student's likelihood of securing a residency spot. If you pass the exam, you do not get an additional chance to retake it to obtain a higher score. It's not like the SAT where you can repeat it to obtain a higher score. I knew my scores weren't the highest, so I decided to pursue an additional my growing interest in research and health disparities by moving to Boston prior to my medical school graduation to pursue a Master's in Public Health at Harvard University. Prior to graduating from medical school, I completed a rotation at the same hospital where I was seen by Dr. McKinley-Grant as a patient. The Chair, Dr. Nigra, told me about his amazing colleague, Dr. Barbara Gilchrest, with whom he trained and was the current Chair of Dermatology at Boston University.

A few weeks after I arrived at Boston University, I met with Dr. Gilchrest to discuss her research on skin aging and my experience as a research fellow at the National Institutes of Health. Dr. Gilchrest invited me to conduct a year of research in her lab after I completed my year at Harvard University. It was those two years that I invested in gaining additional experience that allowed me to be selected for a coveted dermatology residency position in the Boston University/Tufts University Dermatology residency program on my first try. The Dean of Student Affairs at my medical school was not supportive, however. He told me that dermatology was only for students who score in the 99th percentile on the Step 1 exam. I replied, "With all due respect, dermatology is for me as well and I won't allow one exam to rule me out." The strong courage and resolve to pursue my dreams that I developed as a child, which I learned after reading Angela Duckwork's amazing book,

"Grit: The Power of Passion and Perseverance,"[1] is called having a "high grit score." This innate grit stood me well, and provided me with the fortitude and tenacity to develop and execute the needed strategy to gain the edge needed to succeed.

I completed my intern year of residency in Baltimore at the University of Maryland, where I completed medical school. I finished my residency in 2010, and worked at a group practice in Boston until relocating to Western Massachusetts. Looking back, I can see how God opened doors and closed others to bring me here. In 2013, I decided to resign from my position as a staff dermatologist at a large multispecialty group. I prayed at Bible study the evening I left, and asked my family for advice. I knew it was right for my career and future, so I prepared my letter of resignation. I decided to join another practice that wanted to launch their dermatology department, which I would head. I was disappointed a few months later, however, when the new practice informed me they had a hiring freeze and the position I was applying for was no longer available. God was protecting me because a few months later, I learned the practice was folding. I wasn't sure about opening my own practice because I enjoyed the security of a regular paycheck! Many things worked together to make it possible. I found a great location, was able to sign a lease below market value for the first year, and Lenzy Dermatology and Hair Loss Center was born. I was able to get a part-time job covering for a friend on maternity leave so that I could work without a salary until my practice became established. And, with God's great blessing, four years later we have more than 20,000 patients!

---

1   Duckwork, A. (2016). *Grit: The Power of Passion and Perseverance*. Scribner: New York, NY.

WHY I WROTE THIS BOOK

I am grateful for a loving family, for so many opportunities to fulfill my dreams, and the passion I experience every day for the health of my patients. I wish I had unending hours to teach and encourage each one; but since I don't, this book will help to explain some of the most common hair and scalp problems that I see in my practice every day. I want to address the lack of credible information that is available and possibly leading to the often delayed presentation to dermatologists with these problems. I would also like to provide a resource to dermatologists who will be serving the unique needs of patients from various ethnic groups. My passion to educate doesn't stop here, however. I will continue my research and advocacy for cultural competency for every dermatologist, and for my personal quest to give every patient the gift of health, beauty, and healthy hair!

HOW TO READ THIS BOOK

I understand that medical terminology can be overwhelming, especially when someone is experiencing a condition that is affecting their lives physically. The search for answers, or even a hint to what could possibly be happening, can be just as arduous since, as I mentioned before, the internet/social media is full of opinions and "answers". In this book, I have laid out the 16 major types of hair loss and scalp disorders, common scenarios of how they present with a patient's experience with each type of hair loss, the treatment regimens I use, as well as the ones that may be prescribed in general cases. In the Table of Contents, you will see that each chapter is named according to the type of hair loss and the symptoms that come with it. This way, you can quickly identify what you may be experiencing and know the appropriate language to speak when contacting a dermatologist to schedule an appointment.

As you will be able to conclude by reading a few of the chapters, I am a huge advocate for natural hair (haircare without chemicals found in straighteners and some grooming products) and overall health. So, after the 16 major types of hair loss and scalp disorders, I have included two chapters (*Going Natural* and *Nutrition and Hair*) that provide tips on how to care for your hair, as well as your body, that could contribute to the healing process of any hair loss condition you may be experiencing.

I pray that by reading this book, you will feel more knowledgeable and empowered while working with your dermatologist, trichologist, and/or hair stylist to tackle any hair loss issue you may be encountering.

TELOGEN EFFLUVIUM
(EXCESSIVE SHEDDING)

WHAT IS TELOGEN EFFLUVIUM?

Telogen Effluvium (TE) is the clinical name for increased shedding in excess of the normal 100-300 strands daily. TE is the second most common form of hair loss after Androgenetic Alopecia. TE happens when there is a shift in the number of hair follicles from the anagen (or growing) to the telogen (or shedding) phase of the hair cycle.

Healthy hair cycles through three phases. At any given time approximately 85 percent of hairs are in the anagen phase (which lasts two-six years), 10 percent are in the Telogen phase (which lasts three months), and five percent are in a transitional phase called catagen. At the end of the telogen phase, the hair falls out and a new hair will begin the cycle again. In the case of Telogen Effluvium (effluvium means "flow of" in Latin), however, there is a premature shift of hairs from the anagen or growth phase to the catagen and telogen phases, and this disruption to the healthy hair cycle causes shedding in excess of the normal 10 percent or 100-300 strands daily. During peak TE, 500 strands (or more) can be shed daily.

TE usually occurs three months after an "event," which causes disruption of the normal hair cycle. Such "events" include: hormonal changes caused by childbirth, major surgery, rapid weight loss, illness or fever, hypothyroidism, iron deficiency, and chronic stress. There are also nutritional causes of TE, such as: too much vitamin A (which is why it is important to be aware of this when selecting "hair vitamins" as many hair vitamins on the market contain mega doses of vitamin A. Iron, vitamin D, and zinc deficiencies as well as inadequate protein intake are also nutritional causes of excessive shedding (Box 1). TE can also be a side effect of some medicines, including: blood pressure-lowering drugs, blood thinners, cholesterol-lowering drugs, and starting and stopping birth control (Box 1). Though rare, exposure to toxins such as thallium, mercury, and arsenic can also cause TE.

TE affects all ages, ethnicities, and genders. Women may have a greater tendency to experience TE because it commonly follows childbirth. Although it occurs in both genders, women tend to find hair shedding more troublesome than men, and therefore, it is reported more often by women. It can be seen in young babies, the elderly, and all ages in between. With TE, there are no bald spots, and tenderness, redness, or other indications of inflammation are absent. While those affected by TE can experience extreme thinning as a result of severe shedding contrary to many patients' fears, TE does NOT cause complete baldness, as the shedding occurs, the hairs in the anagen-growing phase regrow.

Causes of Telogen Effluvium:

- Endocrine
  - Childbirth, Miscarriage, Abortion
  - Hypo- and Hyperthyroidism
  - Stopping Estrogen-Containing Drugs (Birth control pills)

- "Stressful" events
  - Fever
  - Major Surgery
  - Major Trauma
  - Psychological Stress

- Nutritional
  - Rapid Weight Loss (e.g. "crash dieting")
  - Protein or Calorie Restriction
  - Chronic Iron Deficiency
  - Excessive Vitamin A
  - Vitamin D Deficiency
  - Zinc Deficiency

- Medications
  - Blood Pressure-Lowering Agents: Beta-Blockers (Metoprolol), ACE inhibitors (Captopril)
  - Blood Thinners (Heparin, Warfarin)
  - Cholesterol-Lowering Drugs
  - Colchicine

A PATIENT'S EXPERIENCE WITH TE

Bridget, a 30-year-old woman, came to my office because she noticed her hair falling out and felt that after three weeks of seeing the problem, her hair was losing its density and becoming much thinner. When she shampooed her hair, she noticed that she lost so much of it that the drain was clogged. She even had to buy a new vacuum cleaner because her husband complained that her "hair was everywhere." Bridget frequently wore her hair in a ponytail, and she noticed after three weeks of shedding that her ponytail holder now wrapped around four times instead of the usual two times. Of course, as a woman, this can be very alarming. She even brought in a small bag of hair to show me how much had fallen out over just a few days. Understandably, Bridget was crying as she told me her story. Through her tears and frustration, she looked at me and said, "At this rate, I'm going to be bald soon!"

I assured Bridget that we would identify the cause, and that she most definitely would not go bald. Because her hair loss was diffusely shedding rather than thinning in a pattern on her scalp (as in Androgenetic Alopecia), I suspected that she was experiencing TE but I wanted to be sure. I asked Bridget about her medical history, and she informed me that she wasn't taking any medications and had not dieted recently. She had plenty of energy and she didn't feel cold or mentally fatigued, which was good because these are symptoms that might suggest the need to test thyroid hormone levels. After a few more minutes of questioning, I finally stumbled upon the possible cause of Bridget's condition: birth control. Bridget had been taking birth control pills for about 10 years and had stopped taking them about three months ago.

I examined Bridget's hair and saw diffuse thinning throughout her scalp (see Fig. 2A). I performed a "pull test" in four sections of her scalp, in which I gently tugged on about 25 hairs from the root to the end, which resulted in eight hairs coming out. This is considered a "positive pull test" (more than six hairs or more than three hairs in multiple sections) and demonstrates excessive shedding of the hair consistent with the diagnosis of TE (Fig. 2B).

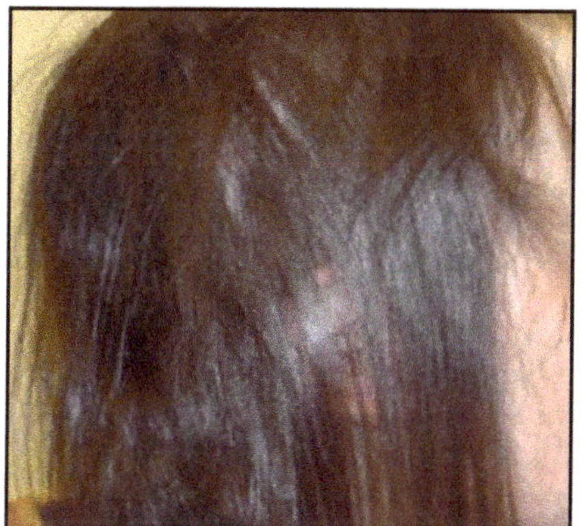

Figure 2A) Diffuse Thinning

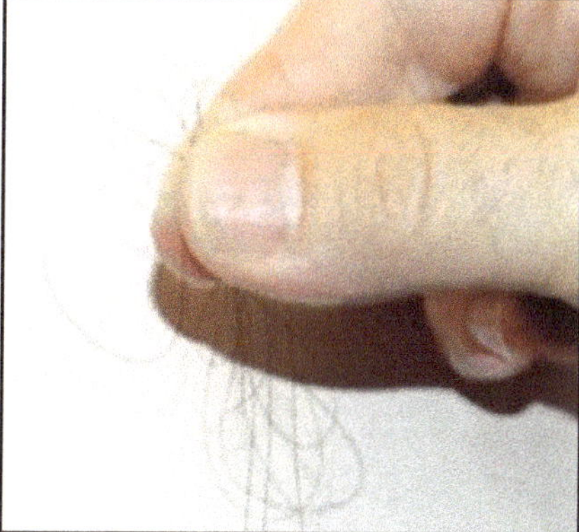

Figure 2B) Positive Pull Test

After explaining the three stages of the hair growth cycle to Bridget, I emphasized that only about 15 percent of the hairs should be in the telogen phase. I used a technique called a trichogram, which allowed me to examine the roots of the hairs with a light microscope to compare the proportion of anagen to telogen hairs. Unfortunately, but not to my surprise, the trichogram revealed that almost 40 percent of Bridget's hairs were in the telogen phase. She was definitely experiencing acute TE, and the only likely trigger factor that we found was stopping her use of birth control pills.

Once I was able to properly pinpoint the cause and type of hair loss Bridget was experiencing, I reassured her once again that, while this condition causes excessive shedding, it does not lead to baldness, and for 90 percent of the patients, the excessive shedding stops in between six to nine months. By then, she could expect her normal hair growth cycle to return and that fortunately, she would experience no scarring or other side effects due to this condition. Ten percent of the time, however, TE can be chronic and persist for more than one year.

TREATMENT OF TE

Very little research has been done to understand TE and after making sure there are no other triggers to remove, the best treatment is the "tincture of time." Although the FDA has not approved any treatments for Acute TE, I mentioned to Bridget that animal studies have found Melatonin to be helpful in decreasing shedding and suggested a trial of 3 mg daily at bedtime, while waiting out the cycle of recovery. Bridget was grateful to know her condition was almost certainly temporary, and with patience, reassurance, and encouragement, she fully recovered in about five months.

Not everyone is as lucky as Bridget, however. In about ten percent of cases, the shedding will not resolve within nine months, and the patient will experience Chronic Telogen Effluvium (CTE). CTE, which usually affects 30- to 60-year-old women, starts abruptly with or without a recognizable initiating factor. An abrupt onset in CTE may be related to a specific event such as childbirth, severe illness, surgery, stress, a crash diet, or various drugs, but often this is not the case and the trigger factor may be obscure. With a gradual onset the cause is often not apparent, but in some cases the shedding may be due to shortened anagen cycles. The duration of the shedding may extend from six months to several years, and the shedding often follows a fluctuating course. The major change that occurs with menopause is the ending of ovarian estrogen production. However, in recent years it has become clear that peri-menopause or the transition to menopause spans a variable period of time when estrogen levels can fluctuate before they decrease to the low stable levels of menopause.[2] This transitional phase occurs on average five years prior to the onset of actual menopause, but can start as early as 10 years prior.[3] Certain environmental exposures such as smoking may hasten the onset of the transitional period. Research data has found that the actual level of estrogen or other hormones may not be correlated with hair shedding but rather a change or variance in levels may lead to CTE.[4] Since hair growth and cycling are both influenced by numerous hormones, growth factors, transcription factors, and cytokines, many of which are known to be modulated by estrogens, it is plausible that an intricate orchestration of these pathways occurs in response to estrogen.[5] Thus, in some women a period of fluctuating estrogen levels during the transition to menopause (albeit in the normal range) could alter hair growth and cycling and elicit episodes of chronic shedding, clinically seen as CTE.

If a particular cause for chronic diffuse hair loss can be identified, such as hypothyroidism or iron deficiency, then suitable treatment should be given. If any drugs are under suspicion as to the cause

---

2   Gold EB. The timing of the age at which natural menopause occurs. *Obstet Gynecol Clin North Am.* 2011;38(3):425–440.

3   Prior, JC. Perimenopause: The complex endocrinology of the menopausal transition. *Endocrine reviews.* 1998;19(4):397–428.

4   Mirmirani P. Hormones and clocks: Do they disrupt the locks? Fluctuating estrogen levels during menopausal transition may influence clock genes and trigger chronic telogen effluvium. *Dermatol Online* J. 2016; May 15;22(5).

5   Ohnemus U, Uenalan M, Inzunza J, Gustafsson JA, & Paus R. The hair follicle as an estrogen tar-get and source. *Endocrine reviews.* 2006;27(6):677–706.

of the shedding, then you can work with your physician to see if it is possible to substitute them with a similar drug that contains fewer risks of causing hair loss. I do not recommend stop taking any drugs on your own without the proper instruction of your physician. If your diet is inadequate, then it should be rectified. If possible, I recommend seeking out dietary sources versus a supplement to enhance your diet with hair healthy foods. If you need additional assistance with this, I recommend my e-book "Dr. Lenzy's Hair Diet: 11 Tips to Achieve Your Best Hair Ever Naturally," which can be purchased at www.LenzyDerm.com.

ANDROGENETIC ALOPECIA
(MALE- & FEMALE-PATTERNED THINNING/BALDNESS)

WHAT IS ANDROGENETIC ALOPECIA?

Androgenetic Alopecia (AGA), also known as male and female pattern hair loss, is the most common form of hair loss in both men and women. Although its exact cause remains unknown, it is related to hormone imbalance, as well as genetic inheritance. The genetic tendency for AGA can be inherited from either the mother or the father, contrary to popular belief that it is only from the maternal side. Women experiencing AGA often describe similar experiences in either parent, uncles, aunts, siblings, or grandparents. A hormonal cause of AGA can be suspected in young women with female pattern thinning, irregular menses, and signs of androgen or male hormone excess, such as excessive facial hair or acne. Although women have less testosterone than men, the same hormonal process occurs in which testosterone is converted to dihydrotestosterone or DHT. DHT is the hormone responsible for the miniaturization of hair follicles.

Female patterns of thinning are different because the presence of female hormones, estrogen and estradiol, and the enzyme that enhances their production, aromatase, mitigates the effects of DHT.[6] Male pattern hair loss or balding tends to start at the temple areas and move toward the crown. In females, the hair loss is more evenly distributed. It is often called the "Christmas Tree pattern" because of its shape from the crown to the front of the scalp.

A PATIENT'S EXPERIENCE WITH AGA

Kathia, a 36-year-old woman, came to my office recently for help with hair loss. Even though I see this problem in my practice on a daily basis, each case has a unique story and there can be one or several underlying problems that finally raise a patient's level of concern to seek help. Kathia noticed changes in the amount of hair falling out about five years ago. She bought special hair growth shampoos, took high-dose biotin and other vitamins for "hair, skin, and nails" recommended on the internet but none of the over-the-counter preparations made a difference. She began combing her hair straight back, since the thinning was at her crown and fairly easy to hide. However, she knew that this only served as a temporary solution.

I carefully examined the thinning area in the crown for any redness or scaling and found none (Fig. 3A). I then used a special handheld magnifying light called a dermatoscope, to more closely

---

6   Otberg N, & Shapiro J. Hair Growth Disorders. In Fitzpatrick's *Dermatology in General Medicine,* (8th Ed.);2012.

examine the root of her hairs (i.e. follicles) in which I saw that some hairs were thinner and smaller than others, demonstrating a process called miniaturization (Fig. 3B). Kathia's scalp was visible through her thinning hair and she also had a linear patch of hair loss in the areas she covered with an adhesive hair replacement unit. Kathia told me that she had been to a "hair loss treatment center" and was told that her diagnosis was Alopecia Areata (another diagnosis we will discuss in Chapter 4). From my years of caring for patients with hair loss, I knew that this was not the type of hair loss that she had. However, I wanted to confirm this by performing a scalp biopsy. A scalp biopsy is the removal of a small, typically 4-mm (less than the size of a pencil eraser) sample of the scalp under local anesthesia (typically lidocaine with epinephrine given with a tiny needle) to make a definitive diagnosis. Usually two stitches or a product called "gel foam" are placed in the area where the biopsy is taken to allow the skin to heal for two weeks.

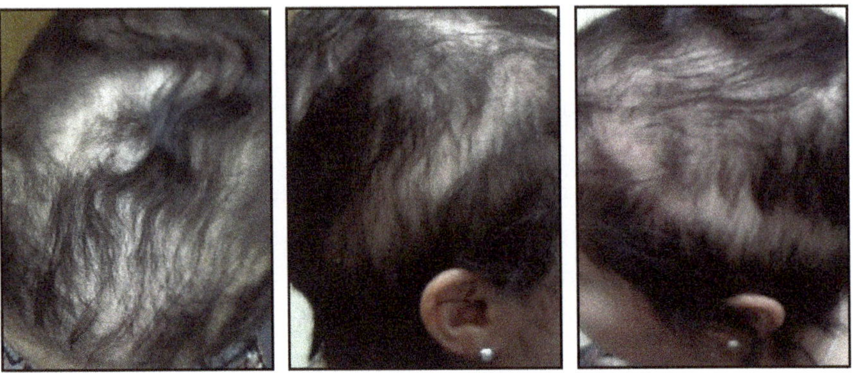

Figure 3A) Female Pattern Thinning (with a Linear Patch of Loss from a Hair Replacement Unit) Before Treatment

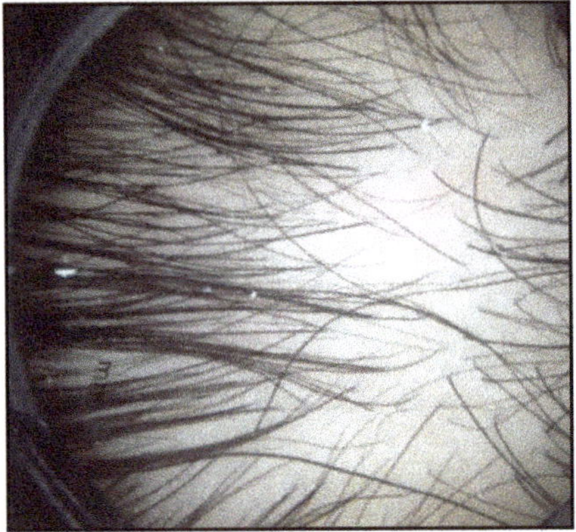

Figure 3B) Trichoscopy of Androgenetic Alopecia with Miniaturization

Kathia's biopsy showed miniaturization and a decrease in the number of terminal hairs (which are the normal hairs that we can see) and an increase in the number of vellus hairs (similar the small hairs that are often visible on the face).

As I discussed my findings with Kathia, I realized she had developed a negative self-esteem and had become withdrawn from her normal social activities because she was embarrassed about her hair. We talked about how the hair loss had affected her everyday functioning, emotions, and concerns about her appearance. I assured her that seeking early treatment was the best way to overcome her hair loss and to return to feeling comfortable in social situations and feeling good about herself.

TREATMENT OF AGA

Minoxidil

I discussed with Kathia several options for treatment. I explained that there is only one FDA-approved treatment for AGA, which is Minoxidil (Rogaine). The Minoxidil 2% solution could be used twice a day, or the 5% foam could be used once a day. The Minoxidil 2% solution is readily available as a liquid or a foam but the solution contains a preservative called propylene glycol, which some people can be sensitive to, causing an itchy scalp. The solution can also cause curly hair that has been heat straightened to revert back to curly. In this case, the treatment can be compounded into an oil or cream that can minimize the effect on thermally straightened hair. After six months of treatment, Kathia was elated to report that her hair was growing back in the thinned areas, and upon examination, we found that the miniaturization of her hair follicles was no longer progressing (Fig. 3C).

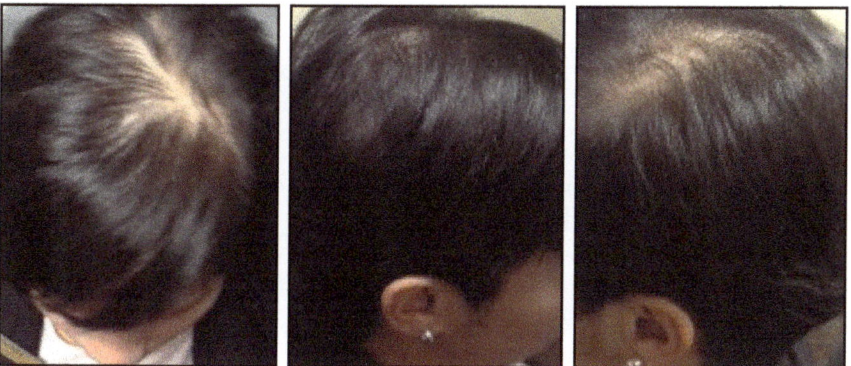

Figure 3C) Female Pattern Thinning after 6 Months of Topical Minoxidil Foam 5%

5-Alpha-Reductase Inhibitors

For men there are two FDA options: Minoxidil or oral Finasteride, 1 mg daily. Inhibitors of the 5-alpha-reductase enzyme, which facilitates the conversion of Testosterone to DHT, like Finasteride or Dutasteride, can be effective in addition to or in lieu of Minoxidil. Patients should be closely monitored for the side effects (notably, sexual side effects in the form of decreased libido and erectile dysfunction rarely occur in less than two percent of participants).[7] It is important to avoid the use of Finasteride in pre-menopausal women who can become pregnant as exposure *in utero* can cause feminization of a male fetus. I do use Finasteride, off-label, in post-menopausal women at a higher dose, namely 2.5 mg or 5 mg, as the 1-mg dose was not effective in clinical trials.[8]

Botanicals

Recently, several botanicals (or natural alternatives) have been published as alternatives to Finateride for blocking DHT, the hormone responsible for the miniaturization seen in AA (Table 2).[9]

---

7   Kaufman KD, Olsen EA, et al. Finasteride in the treatment of men with androgenetic alopecia. Finasteride Male Pattern Hair Loss Study Group. *J Am Acad Dermatol.* 1998 Oct;39(4 Pt 1):Vol 39:578–589.

8   Camacho FM, Randall VA, Price VH. (2000) *Hair and Its Disorders: Biology Pathology and Management.* Martin Dunitz: London.

9   Rondanelli M, Perna, S, Peroni G, Guido D. A bibliometric study of scientific literature in Scopus on botanicals for treatment of androgenetic alopecia. *J Cosmet Dermatol.* 2016;15:120–130.

Table 1

Camelia sensis (Green tea) Epigallocatechin gallate (EGCG), the main flavonoid in Camelia sinensis, shows potent inhibition of 5-alpha-reductase.
Carthamus tinctorius (Safflower), is a plant species that is widely used both in the food industry (as an additive, flavoring, etc.) and in the herbal industry
Puerariae Flos (the flowers of the plant Pueraria thomsonii) due to its potent inhibitor of 5-alpha-reductase, reducing Dihydrotestosterone (DHT) which is responsible for miniaturization of hair follicle miniaturization
Red ginseng, the steamed root of *Panax ginseng* has a long history use as a medicinal herb in East Asia and inhibits the DHT-induced androgen receptor transcription promoting hair growth
Ginkgo biloba plant, rich in Quercetin, is a bioflavonoid with anti-inflammatory properties
Serenoa repens (Saw palmetto) is a natural Dihydrotestosterone (DHT) blocker
Rosmarinus officinalis, a culinary aromatic and medicinal plant, is very rich in polyphenols and flavonoids with high antioxidant properties
Bee venom, inhibits the expression of the *SRD5A2* gene, which encodes a type II 5-alpha-reductase that plays a major role in the conversion of testosterone into dihydrotestosterone.

Nutraceuticals

There are several formulated combinations of botanical ingredients, which are termed "nutracueticals." Viviscal (OTC) and Viviscal Professional Strength (sold by physician offices and beauty professionals) are dietary supplements with the active ingredient marine complex formulation, which was originally developed in the late 1980s in Scandinavia. The first clinical trial published in 1992 was found to significantly increase the number of terminal hairs (which are the thicker hairs that we can see versus the vellus or "baby hairs," which are present on our face) in women with thinning hair. The professional contains the 475 mg of the marine complex while the OTC strength contains 450 mg. Viviscal also contains Apple Extract Powder (Pyocyanidin B-2), which has been shown to increase hair density and diameter. It contains a 100 mcg Biotin vs mega doses of 5,000-10,000 mcg present in many standalone Biotin supplements and other supplements, which often cause acne as an associated side effect. Vitamin C, which is an anti-oxidant, is believed to protect hair and skin from free radicals. L-Cystine and L-Methionine, which are essential amino acids. In the clinical trial, Viviscal users saw an 80 percent increase in the number of terminal hair (which are the thicker hairs that we can see vs the vellus or "baby hairs" which are present on our face, for example).

Nutrafol is a newer nutraceutical, which targets several possible triggers of hair thinning, including DHT with saw palmetto, which is a plant-based DHT blocker. Ashwagandha root (also known as Indian ginseng), which has been used for hundreds of years in ayurvedic medicine, has been shown to have anti-stress effects by decreasing cortisol and inflammatory C-reactive protein and improve resistance to stress. It also contains Curcumin, a component of the golden spice turmeric, which is an antioxidant and has shown anti-inflammatory effects in a number of anti-inflammatory diseases, including cancer, cardiovascular disease, arthritis, and skin conditions, including vitiligo and psoriasis. It is suspected that it may help to optimize the immune system and fight many inflammatory molecules that slow hair growth.

Microneedling and Platelet-Rich Plasma

Microneedling and Platelet-Rich Plasma (PRP) treatment are in-office treatments, which can be done alone or in combination. Microneedling is a procedure where a microneedling device (like the SkinPen, dermaroller, or the cosmopen) creates multiple microchannels that can increase penetration of complimentary medications such as Minoxidil or platelet-rich plasma into the deeper layer of scalp called the dermis. Needles (1.5 mm in size) are gently rolled over the affected areas of the scalp until mild redness is noted weekly for a series of sessions. A numbing cream can be applied one to two hours prior to the procedure, which takes about 20-25 minutes. Patients are typically advised to continue with their ongoing therapy with finasteride and Minoxidil. Microneedling stimulates hair regrowth by the following mechanisms: release of growth factors (platelet-derived growth factor and epidermal growth factor) through the wound healing process; activation of stem cells in the hair bulge area, and overexpression of hair growth-related genes.[10] Activated PRP appears to promote differentiation of stem cells into hair follicle cells. PRP prolongs the anagen phase through increased expression of growth factors and increases cell survival by stopping cell death called apoptosis. A

10 Kachhawa D, Vats G, et al. A split head study of efficacy of placebo versus platelet-rich plasma injections in the treatment of androgenic alopecia. *J Cutan Aesthet* Surg. 2017;10:86–89.

significant increase in hair density was noted (from mild to significant improvement) in multiple studies (Fig. 3A - Fig. 3C).[11]

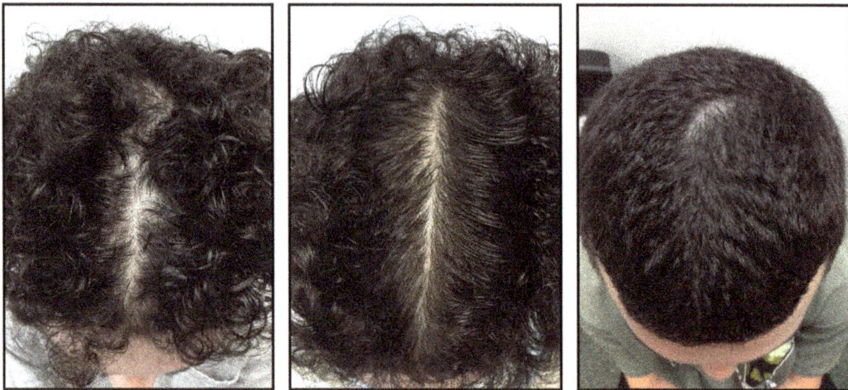

Figure 3D) Left, Before PRP Treatment Middle, After 6 Months Right, After 1 Year

Low-Level Light Therapy

A relatively new and innovative therapy for AGA involves the use of low-level laser/light treatment. Paradoxical hair growth has occurred in patients undergoing laser hair removal when low energy fluences were used. Light-emitting diode (LED) wavelengths are known to be absorbed by the mitochondria within the cells, which produce increased adenosine triphosphate (ATP), leading to increased cellular signaling related to hair growth. One theory suggests an increase in blood flow in the dermal papilla, inflammation improvement, and growth factor production. A recent study of various wavelengths of LED demonstrated stimulation of outer root sheath cells and inhibition of cell death via the Wnt5a-β-catenin and extracellular-signal-regulated kinase (ERK)

11 Shah KB, Shah AN, et al. A comparative study of microneedling with platelet-rich plasma plus topical minoxidil (5%) and topical minoxidil (5%) alone in androgenetic alopecia. *Int J Trichol.* 2017;9:14–18.

signaling pathways, which upregulates genes responsible for cell proliferation in hair cells and causing anagen re-entry. Several clinical trials examine whether low-level laser devices increase terminal hair density in both men and women with pattern hair loss.

Several studies have demonstrated a statistically significant increase in hair density between lasercomb- and placebo-treated subjects. Additionally, a higher percentage of lasercomb-treated subjects reported overall improvement in the thickness and fullness of hair in self-assessment, compared with placebo-treated subjects. Another study was designed to examine the efficacy and safety of a helmet-type, home-use LLLT device emitting wavelengths of 630, 650, and 660 nm versus a placebo device for 18 minutes daily. After 24 weeks of treatment, the LLLT group showed significantly greater hair density than the placebo device group. Average hair diameter improved statistically significantly more in the LLLT group than in the placebo device group. There were no serious adverse reactions were detected.

Hair Restoration Surgery

For those who do not improve with medical or laser therapy, hair transplantation is an option. Generally, this procedure is done by taking hair from the "donor" area in the occipital scalp, and transplanting them to the thinning areas in the crown and frontal scalp. Anywhere from 5,000 to 7,000 follicular units can be transplanted in one session, and multiple sessions can be performed until the desired of hair transplanted has been achieved. Performing this procedure on African Americans can be more challenging compared with other ethnicities due to curved hair follicles, lower hair density (which is the number of hairs per square centimeter), and a higher risk of keloid formation (an excessive growth of scar tissue). Therefore, it is a good idea for patients with a family history of keloid formation to have a test transplant before full-scale grafting is performed.

Hair Replacement Units

Patients who do not respond to medical therapies may wish to choose a practical solution by selecting an appropriate hair replacement unit called a "scalp prosthesis" (the medical term for a custom wig unit) to help them look and feel their best. I do recommend a custom unit as an investment due to the ability to have it made for the most accurate fit, as an ill-fitted unit can provide unwanted stress on the edges and possibly contribute to traction alopecia. A custom unit can be colored and cut in a style that will be the most flattering by a trained hair loss specialist stylist or trichologist. Some insurance companies may provide partial coverage of a unit with a prescription from your dermatologist for a scalp prosthesis. Typically, you pay for the unit up front and submit your receipt to the insurance company for reimbursement. I recommend checking on your insurance plan's coverage prior to starting the process.

With all of the medical, natural, and surgical developments, a dermatologist who specializes in hair loss can provide you with a plethora of options based on your preferences, which can help to prevent further progression and even help to achieve significant regrowth in many cases. The key, as with all forms of hair loss, is the importance of an early diagnosis.

ALOPECIA AREATA
(BALD SPOTS)

WHAT IS ALOPECIA AREATA?

Alopecia Areata (AA) is an autoimmune form of hair loss in which the immune system makes a "mistake" and produces a type of T-cell (CD8+) that "attacks" the hair follicle, resulting in circular patches of hair loss. AA is not a result of taking medication or a symptom of illness. Most individuals with AA are otherwise healthy other than the hair loss. It is not contagious and is not a condition solely caused by "stress," as I have sometimes heard. The lifetime risk of developing AA is 1.7 percent, and the risk is the same for all ethnic groups.

AA sometimes occurs in patients with other autoimmune conditions. A medical center in Boston reviewed 2,115 patients with AA and reported that patients with AA have a higher occurrence of other autoimmune diseases, including thyroid disease (14.6%), Type 1 diabetes (11.1%), and inflammatory bowel syndrome

(6.3%). AA is the most common form of hair loss found in children, and almost one-half of cases are in patients younger than 20 years of age.

AA can occur in different subtypes: patchy (a single or multiple typically circular patched of hair loss (Fig. 4A); ophiasis (isolated loss of a band of hair on the sides and back or the parietal and occipital scalp (Fig. 4B, left and right); barbae (circular patches of hair loss in the beard area (Fig. 4C); Alopecia Totalis (AT) (total hair loss on the entire scalp) and Alopecia Universalis (AU) (hair loss over the entire body, including the eyebrows, eyelashes, and body hair.

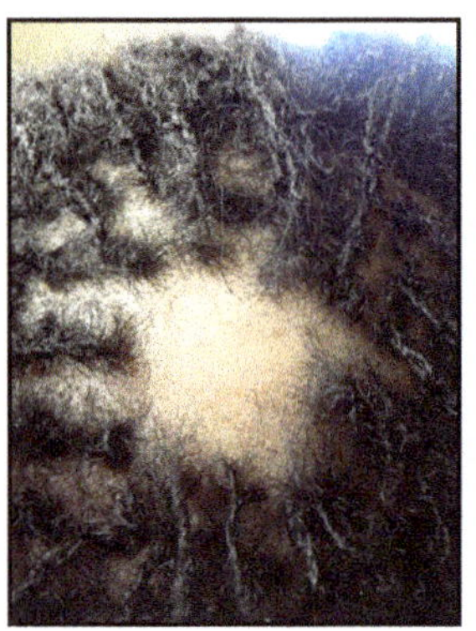

Figure 4A) Patchy Alopecia Areata

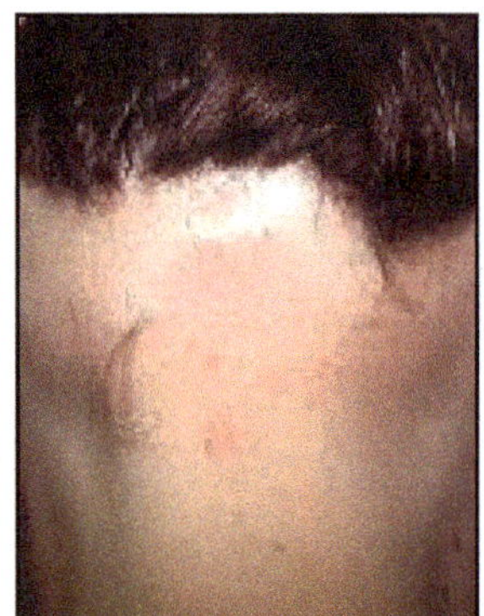

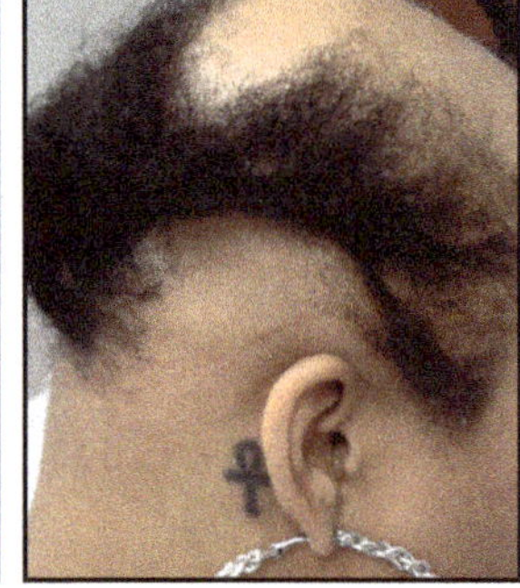

Figure 4B) Ophiasis Pattern

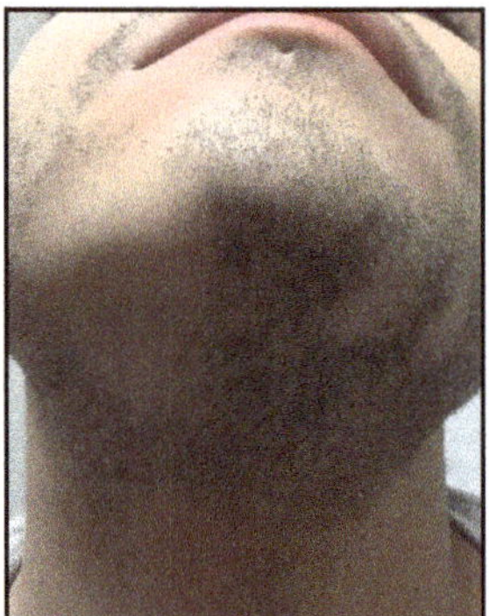

Figure 4C) Alopecia Barbae

A PATIENT'S EXPERIENCE WITH AA

Leland, a 25-year-old male, came to my office because of rapid complete hair loss on the scalp over a four-month period. Leland had a history of AA as a child, with episodes of round quarter-sized bald spots on the scalp. His first experience lasted for a few months when he was five years old, and again when he was seven years old. The present complete hair loss he was experiencing, or AT, followed a stressful divorce.

Leland exhibited one of the less common subtypes of AA. About 80 percent of patients have only one round patch, usually on the scalp. Twelve percent have two patches, and 7.7 percent have multiple bald spots. In males, the beard is involved in 28 percent of patients, and more than one area can be affected at once. Only about five percent of patients experience the total hair loss on the scalp that Leland was experiencing (AT), and about one percent experience a loss of all body hair, AU. When the hair loss is isolated to the back (occipital) and sides (parietal) of the scalp, called the Ophiasis pattern, it is particularly difficult to treat.

Leland blamed his rapid hair loss on the stress in his life, but AA is associated with a major life event only about 15 percent of the time. Most patients do not have a triggering factor present. Leland mentioned his five-year-old niece who had come to see me about a year prior to this visit. Unlike Leland's childhood experience, she began with only a few bald spots on her scalp, but rapidly progressed to AT. After talking to her and her parents, we agreed that she was not under any added stress at all. AA, though some families are genetically predisposed, can happen to anyone with no warning or particular reason. I prescribed a topical cortisone called Clobetasol to decrease the inflammation (the T-cells) around the follicles for Leland's niece, which her mother applied to her scalp daily for three weeks, then she took one week off, and repeated. Leland reported that her hair had grown back to normal, and he was hoping his condition would resolve just as quickly. He wanted to know how soon he could expect his hair to grow back, but unfortunately, there is no way to predict how long or to what extent this type of hair loss will persist. If it affects less than 50% of the scalp, spontaneous regrowth will probably occur within several months. Leland, however, had a lower expected response rate, or prognosis, because he had experienced AA as a child, and his current episode was much more extensive.

TREATMENT OF AA

In spite of the unpredictable outcome, I assured Leland that his condition would not affect his overall health, and that we would treat the problem aggressively for three months to see if regrowth would occur, and described the maintenance treatment we would consider. My first line of treatment in AA is a potent prescription topical steroid cream that is applied to the affected area daily for three weeks, followed by a week of rest, then three additional weeks of treatment. Leland was treated with the combination therapy of topical steroids and steroid injections, called Kenalog injections, which are able to penetrate to the deeper layers of the scalp every six to eight weeks until the desired amount of regrowth occurs. A very small needle (the same ones that diabetics use to inject insulin) is used to inject the medication into the affected areas with approximately 1 cm between injection sites. The combination therapy of injections with the topical cortisone is more effective than using topical cortisone alone. When hair regrowth begins, I recommend off-label treatment with Minoxidil 5% foam to the affected area daily. Minoxidil stimulates the hair follicle to produce a thicker strand of hair, and prolongs the growing, or anagen stage, of the hair cycle. Though Leland grew sparse vellus hair during treatment, it fell out within several weeks after he stopped treatment. He decided to wait and see if any spontaneous regrowth would occur before considering the topical irritant therapy.

Irritant Contact Therapy

A second line of therapy may be used with chronic severe AA to create skin irritation in the area with the hopes of causing the body's immune system to mount an immune response. Although the exact mechanism is not clear, it is believed that the T-cells attacking the follicle shift to the skin because of the irritation. A very dilute solution of irritant in the form of Squaric Acid or DPCP is applied to the affected area, and each week the concentration of the solution is increased until it produces redness and mild itching. Once the proper concentration is determined and until there is complete regrowth, patients can experience swollen lymph nodes, and may also notice skin discoloration. Success rates vary from 17 percent to 75 percent, depending on the type of AA, the age of the patient, and the length of time the patient has had symptoms. Although this treatment has been in use for two decades, it is not FDA approved. There is about three months from the start of therapy to evidence of re-growth, and treatment should be continued for at least one year. The relapse rate after stopping therapy is about 62 percent.

Systemic Treatments

Oral steroids such as prednisone can be used in cases of rapid hair loss in an attempt to stop rapid progression, but they are not the treatment of choice because of side effects with long-term use and the high incidence of relapse when the steroids are discontinued. Exciting new treatments are on the horizon for AA, including medications, which block a pathway called Janus kinase inhibitors (or JAK inhibitors), called Tofacitinib or Ruxolitinib. Tofacitinib was recently featured on the nightly news when a patient with psoriasis who happened to have Alopecia Universalis for many years, was treated with Tofacitinib and experienced complete hair regrowth of his scalp and body hair as well as the eyelashes and eyebrows within eight months. For this reason, the article, which published in the Journal of Investigative Dermatology, was aptly titled, "Killing Two Birds with One Stone: Oral Tofacitinib Reverses Alopecia Universalis in a Patient with Plaque Psoriasis."[12] Subsequently, numerous similar articles have been published describing amazing cases of complete AA regrowth within months of treatment with JAK inhibitors.[13] Two open-label clinical trials and multiple case series of adolescent and adult patients and case reports have been published. Hair loss appears to recur with treatment discontinuation.[14] Recently, two studies showed successful treatment of severe AA, AT, and AU over a period of up to 18 months using Tofacitinib. In 65 adults with either AT or AU with a duration of current episode of alopecia of less than 10 years or severe AA, 77 percent of patients achieved some hair regrowth, with 58 percent achieving 50 percent improvement and 20 percent achieving 90 percent improvement in their Severity of Alopecia Tool or SALT score. Hair regrowth was reduced in

---

12 Craiglow BG, King BA. Killing two birds with one stone: oral tofacitinib reverses alopecia univer-salis in a patient with plaque psoriasis. *J Invest Dermatol.* 2014 Dec;134(12):2988–2990.

13 Liu LY, Craiglow BG, et al. Tofacitinib for the treatment of severe alopecia areata and variants: A study of 90 patients. *J Am Acad Dermatol.* 2017 Jan;76(1):22–28.

14 Damsky W, King BA. JAK inhibitors in dermatology: The promise of a new drug class. *J Am Acad Dermatol.* 2017;76:736–744.

patients with AT and AU with duration greater than 10 years.[14] In adolescents (12-17 years old) with severe AA, AT, and AU, treatment with Tofacitinib resulted in a 93% average change in SALT score from baseline after an average of 6.5 months of treatment.

These medications are not yet FDA approved for AA but are in the midst of Phase III clinical trials. It is important to note that the JAK inhibitors are not without potential side effects, which must be considered prior to treatment. A concern with JAK inhibitors is a theoretical increased risk for malignancy because suppressing the immune system could dampen the body's ability to fight against tumor development. Initial studies of Tofacitinib in transplant patients showed that approximately one percent of patients treated with Tofacitinib developed post-transplant malignancies.[15] However, in these studies patients were treated with much higher doses of Tofacitinib (10-30 mg, twice daily) than is typically used in AA (5 mg, twice daily) and in combination with other immunosuppressive agents, which increases the overall amount of immune system suppression. An increased risk of cancers has not been seen when Tofacitinib is used to treat inflammatory disorders, such as rheumatoid arthritis and psoriasis, which uses a similar dosing as AA. Longer term studies, however, will more definitively answer this question.

---

15 Damsky W, King BA. JAK inhibitors in dermatology: The promise of a new drug class. *J Am Acad Dermatol.* 2017;76:736–744.

A MOTHER'S JOURNEY OF HOPE THROUGH AA

Sandra Dunn

Right before my daughter Arianna turned five, I noticed a small patch of hair was missing from her scalp. Blessed with long, thick, beautiful hair, my daughter loved wearing her hair in different styles. The newly missing patch of hair was making it difficult to put her hair up without exposing the missing patch. Concerned by the sudden loss of hair, I made an appointment for Arianna with her primary care doctor (PCP). Her doctor ran some tests, including blood work, to check her blood counts. After passing all of her tests her PCP suggested we see a dermatologist. We ended up at UCONN in the dermatology department. During our initial consultation, they diagnosed Arianna with AA. They told us not to worry and that her hair would likely grow back. They did recommend that we follow-up with Dr. Lenzy, a dermatologist who specializes in treatment of hair. They told us if anyone knew what to do, she would.

I immediately made an appointment with Dr. Lenzy. After hearing the diagnosis, my husband googled hair loss in children and AA was the first article that popped up. We went through some of the different images and noticed many of the children's photos looked just like Arianna's hair. It gave us some relief to know we were not the only one's experiencing this situation but we still had some anxiety about the time frame and rate of regrowth. I don't have any other family members with AA but my husband has a cousin with lupus who also has AA. That was the extent of our personal exposure or knowledge of AA. My husband continued educating our family on AA through the internet as we waited on our October appointment with Dr. Lenzy.

The day came and I took Arianna to meet with Dr. Lenzy. She walked into the room and immediately put us at ease. She was very friendly and personable. Just as important, however, she was extremely knowledgeable. She talked with us about the different treatments available – the side effects as well as the benefits. With my daughter being so young, Dr. Lenzy wanted to ensure the benefits would far outweigh any side effects. She started us on a topical steroid cream and within a few weeks we saw regrowth of the hair. We were so happy! Unfortunately, our success did not last long. Within six months of the diagnosis, Arianna went from missing one patch of hair to being completely bald.

I sent Arianna and my older daughter to my sister's house to stay for a few weeks over the summer. Before she left I put braided ponytails in her hair. When she came back from her visit, all of her hair had pretty much fallen out. She had a couple of the ponytails hanging on by a few strains of hair. Up until this day, my daughter had been pretty hopeful and optimistic. But the thought of being completely bald was more than her little heart could handle.

"Arianna, I'm going to have to cut off the rest of your hair." I said to her as I approached with scissors in my hand from the kitchen drawer.

Arianna started to cry and took off running to her room. Through her tears she was screaming, "No! No! No, mommy, please don't cut my hair!"

That moment was really difficult for me as a mom. It was really tough. I cried with her and tried my best to just comfort her. I held her in my arms, dropping the scissors and weeping with her. So many fears went through my mind. My daughter is one of my most precious gifts and now because of AA, I was feeling a bit hopeless and unable to help her. What will the other children say? How will they treat her? Will her hair grow back? When will it grow back? She's just a baby. Why is this happening to her? Many thoughts tracked through my mind but the biggest question I had was would my five year old daughter be ok? I didn't have the answer and only time would tell.

After a little time and with tears streaming down both of our cheeks, I picked up the scissors and cut off the remaining braids – holding on to her scalp by strands – from my daughter's head. She was now completely bald. Six months ago, she had a full head of long, beautiful, seemingly healthy hair. Now, she had lost it all. Would she still be the little girl with the big smile and overflowing self-confidence? Hair is important to the confidence of girl's self-esteem, right? Well, before our family went through this battle with hair loss and AA, I would've said yes. But now, I know otherwise.

A few weeks after Arianna went completely bald we were all sitting in the living room watching television and a little girl who was bald like Arianna appeared on the screen. Everyone's attention was focused on the girl. She shared her story of cancer and the pain she was going through. After hearing her story, my daughter crawled up in my lap, hugged me, and said, "Mom, I'm so glad I have Alopecia Areata and not cancer."

I cried a bit but this time the tears fell because of relief. I, too, was glad Arianna's baldness was from AA and not a life-threatening illness such as cancer. I also cried a bit for the mother of that little girl because I imagined her pain was even greater than mine—not only has she dealt with her daughter's baldness but the heart-wrenching fact that her little girl might not be here with her in the foreseeable future. I held both of my girls a little longer and a little tighter that night before going to bed. For the first time, I was thankful for AA.

Since Arianna started her journey with AA, we have used different treatment options. At times we have seen regrowth only to have it all fall out again. There are a few other options we could try but Dr. Lenzy does not suggest we do them right now because the side effects – overworking the liver and kidney – are too risky for Arianna's age. My husband and I agree with her assessment and at this point have stopped treatment. We are still hopeful that full regrowth will happen but we now pour most of our energy into giving our girls a healthy, happy home environment to blossom into beautifully confident girls. So far, we believe and have evidence that we are doing a great job.

On the first day of school last year I received a phone call from the school's principal, Mr. G. I was bit nervous, as all of those fears of bullying and being mistreated came flooding back to my mind. My anxiety quickly turned into a smile as the principal shared his favorite first day of school story with me.

The principal was standing in the bus circle greeting all of the students as they walked off the bus to enter school on the first day. There were lots of giggles with a few timid students mixed in the bunch. As the third bus pulled up and began to unload, Mr. G. noticed Arianna walking towards him with a look of determination in her eyes.

"Good Morning, Mr. G."

"Good Morning, Arianna."

"I know hats are not allowed in school but I have Alopecia Areata, and I have to wear this hat."

He told me that he was tickled by her "matter-of-fact" attitude but was simultaneously grateful that she had the courage to speak her heart.

Mr. G went on to tell me that he was very proud of Arianna and that he told her she could wear her hat and if anyone – teachers or students – gave her a hard time to come directly to his office and let him know.

I was proud of her and felt so blessed to have her under the care of Mr. G. while she was at school. Many of her classmates have embraced Arianna and her hats. During a field trip to the apple patch, her hat got stuck on a tree branch as the class walked by. The teacher quickly grabbed the hat down and put it back on Arianna's head. Arianna was a bit embarrassed for the rest of the field trip and stayed glued to the teacher the rest of the time. However, the next day her classmates were extra careful and watched out for her. One of her classmates saw that her hat wasn't all the way down and told her right away. Later that day on the playground another girl pulled her hat back down when she noticed it was not snug on her head.

Overtime, we have learned as a family not to make a big deal of AA. Arianna's confidence in who she is despite AA has helped us all. I am hopeful that a cure will be found but until then I am dedicated to raising Arianna to be confident and to love herself whether or not she has a full head of hair.

TRICHORRHEXIS NODOSA
(BREAKAGE)

WHAT IS TRICHORRHEXIS NODOSA?

Trichorrhexis Nodosa (TN), the clinical name for hair breakage, is a condition in which weak points along the hair shaft cause the hair to break more easily at those points. TN can be inherited as a dominant trait in some families, caused by an underlying disorder, like hypothyroidism or iron deficiency, or it can be triggered by certain hair styling and/or chemical use. In women, TN can affect hair of the scalp and the pubic area; in men, it can affect the beard and mustache.

While TN affects individuals of all ethnicities, it is more common among people of Afro-Caribbean descent often due to hairstyling practices. In 2005, the L'Oreal Institute for Ethnic Hair surveyed 1,200 women of African American, Asian, Chinese, and Mexican descent, and reported their findings in the International Journal of Dermatology.[16] They found that an overwhelming 96 percent of

---

16 Bryant H, Porter C, & Yang G. Curly hair: Measured differences and contributions to breakage. *Int J Dermatol.* 2012 Nov;51 Suppl 1:8–11, 9–13.

African Americans reported experiencing hair breakage, and 23 percent said it was their "biggest hair problem." Pertaining to the protective cuticle, differences in cuticle spacing, and the number of layers have been found based on race. Increasing space between cuticle layers has been shown in Caucasian vs Asian vs African hair.[17] In a study of Japanese and Caucasian hairs, a smaller cuticle spacing was smaller for Japanese hair as well as more cuticle layers.[18] One may speculate that the tighter the layers and the greater they are in number, the greater protection they provide.

The L'Oreal study concluded that African American hair is more fragile due to structural differences as well as grooming habits and practices. The grooming habits they observed in those with healthy hair were using less force when grooming, less combing, larger tooth combs, air drying rather than heat drying, and less frequent relaxer use. TN also manifests itself differently in African Americans and Caucasians. For African Americans, the hair usually breaks off at the scalp before it has a chance to grow long, whereas people of Caucasian descent usually experience issues with breakage at the end of the hair shaft in the form of hair thinning and split ends.

---

17 Tang D, Porter C, Barbarat P, et al. African-American hair damage characterization and quantifica-tion. Proceedings of 13th International Hair Science Symposium, Potsdam, Germany, 2003.

18 Takahashi T, Hayashi R, Okamoto M, & Inoue S. Morphology and properties of Asian and Cau-casian hair. *J Cosmet Sci.* 2006;57:327–338.

A PATIENT'S EXPERIENCE WITH TN

Victoria is a 35-year-old African American female who came for an office visit with what she called "broken hair with severe split ends". She had been noticing for months that her hair seemed brittle and had broken off in different lengths. At the beginning of the summer, she had also started to notice a problem with dandruff so she used a selenium shampoo for two months with improvement. However, this still wasn't solving her breakage issue.

While a congenital form of TN can be inherited as a dominant trait in some   families, Victoria had no extended family members who had experienced hair breakage. Growing up she wore her hair short in a natural style or in braids. She felt her energy level was high and had no history of anemia or thyroid deficiency, so knowing these things allowed me to rule out congenital TN or suspicion for any underlying thyroid or anemia cause of breakage.

After further probing to try and pinpoint the possible causes of Victoria's condition, we eventually got around to the discussion of her hair care routine. This is where I discovered that just like many of us women, Victoria had been having lots of fun experimenting with her hair. She had been lightening her hair to a light brown for the past two years and because of her love of sunbathing and swimming at her condominium community, her hair was exposed to chlorine up to three to four times per week. Her daily styling routine consisted of shampooing, blow drying, flat ironing, and back combing to create more "lift," combined with gel to give her hair the volume she enjoyed.

Upon examination, Victoria showed signs of both physical and chemical trauma to her hair. Just as she had mentioned, I noticed she had hair of different lengths, which were more pronounced on the side she slept on, at the edges of her scalp, at the nape of her neck, and individual hairs were frayed or split at the ends. Fraying can easily be observed by examining the end of the hair against a piece of paper with contrasting color. Because Victoria's hair was light in color, I examined her hair against a black card. If you can imagine two make-up brushes that have been pushed together so the bristles fan out, that's what the ends looked like (Fig. 5A). Her hair was also dry and dull with breakage noted throughout her scalp (Fig. 5B).

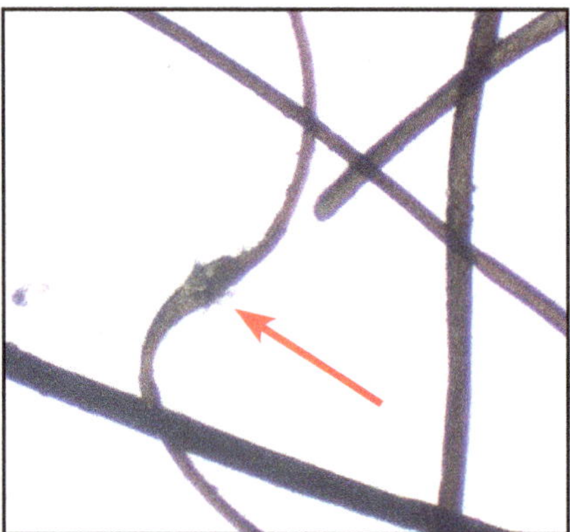

**Figure 5A) Trichorrhexis Nodosa Node
(red arrow, under the microscope)**

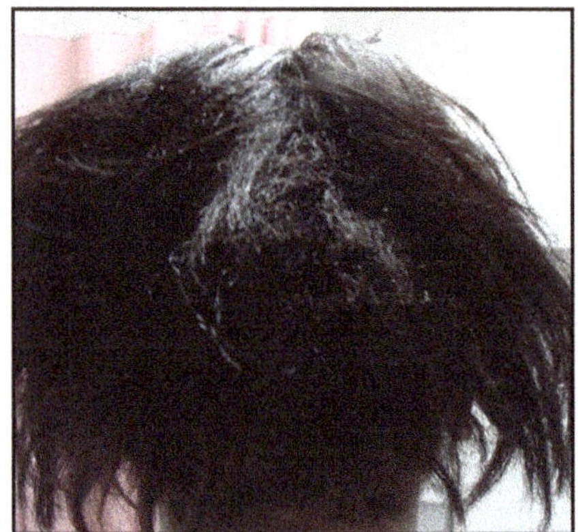
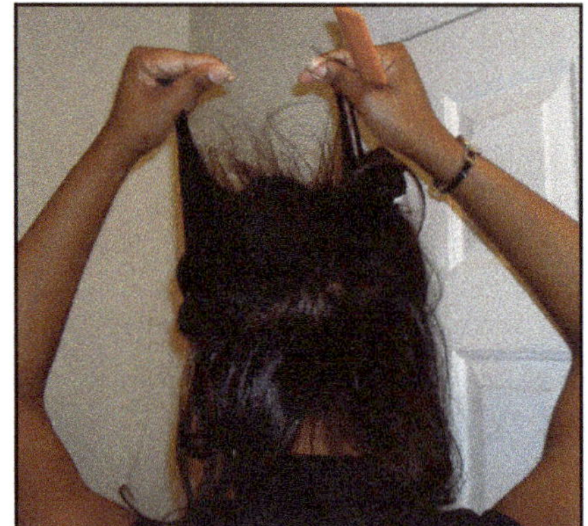

Figure 5B) Trichorrhexis Nodosa

Dullness can result from damage to the hair's outer layer, also known as the cuticle. The cuticle is made of cells that overlap along the length of the hair fiber and it protects the inner cortex, which contains the more fragile hair fibers. The cuticle is damaged during bleaching and other chemical processing. In order for these chemical processes to take effect, the cuticle must be opened up so the bleach can remove hair pigment. When these chemicals are used for an extended period of time or in high concentration, the cuticle can be stripped away, causing the hair to appear dull and become dry and frizzy. In Victoria's case, there were multiple chemical traumas to her hair: two years of bleaching, harsh shampoo, and a good amount of chlorine from swimming. Add on exposure to ultraviolet (UV) light, excessive heat styling, back combing/brushing and an alcohol based gel and you have the ultimate set up for hair damage in the form of TN.

Hair shafts affected by TN contain small white nodes at irregular intervals, which represent the places where cuticle damage has occurred and the inner layer of fibers has frayed. Using extremely high heat will heat and expand the water pushing spaces in the hair fiber. This condition is called "bubble hair," and the weakened hair is more likely to break off.[19]

---

19 Detwiler SP, Carson JL, et al. Bubble hair. Case caused by an overheating hair dryer and reproduc-ibility in normal hair with heat. *J Am Acad Dermatol.* 1994;30:54–60.

TREATMENT OF TN

The best way to nurse your hair back to health after dealing with severe breakage is simply, gentle and natural grooming. It is important to avoid excessive manipulation, chemical hair color, relaxers, and high heat. If hair is fragile and showing signs of breakage, it is also important to avoid braids and locks.

Because of Victoria's use of harsh shampoo, while spending extra time in the sun, she needed to use hair products that were gentle and could help her to restore the moisture stripped away from her hair. Many shampoos contain sulfates, which are detergents that effectively cleanse the hair and scalp. But while they do a fantastic job of cutting through the product build-up, they can contribute to increased dryness, which in Victoria's case, can further contribute to the breakage and damage she's already experiencing. Because of this, I recommended Victoria invest in a sulfate-free moisturizing shampoo that would allow gentle cleansing, as well as deep conditioning steam treatments and provide more moisture during her styling process.

Shea butter contains vitamins A and E, and is a natural sunscreen and hair protectant, which could help to shield Victoria's hair from the swimming pool salt and chlorine that had previously dried out her hair. For swimmers, I recommend applying a pre-shampoo treatment called a "pre-poo" to effectively coat the hair prior to exposure to chlorine or salt water.

One of the unfortunate effects of TN is that breakage cannot be fully repaired and it may be necessary to cut off the severely damaged hair. When the breakage involves more than 50% of the scalp, I typically recommend cutting the hair all to one length due the difficulty in managing hairs of various lengths. Victoria is one of those brave people who decided to do so. She discontinued bleaching her hair and transitioned from the braids she had been wearing to what many in the natural haircare community refer to as the "Big Chop," which consists of cutting off the damaged hair and wearing a TWA (Teenie Weenie Afro, see Fig. 1) in an effort to start fresh and grow hair back that's strong and healthy. Victoria selected a sulfate-free moisturizing shampoo to use weekly as well as a "pre-poo" moisturizing treatment to add moisture and softness. Pre-pooing is a very simple, but effective step done before shampooing your hair that protects your hair from being stripped of its natural oils and moisture. You can create your own pre-poo by using a few tablespoons of jojoba oil, or a blend of oils. There are also several commercially available oil treatments that contain avocado and argan oil, which can be used.

To perform a pre-poo, perform the following steps:

1. Put your oil in a small container and place it in hot water for a few minutes. Heating the oil helps it to open your hair cuticles to allowing better penetration.

2. Massage the warm oil into your scalp for two to three minutes, then rub the oil down the shaft of your hair, out to the ends. Only a small amount of oil is needed to get the desired result.

3. Cover your hair with a plastic shower cap. Then, submerge a towel in very hot water, squeeze out the excess water and wrap your head (over the shower cap) with the hot towel for 30 minutes. Alternatively, you can sit under a steamer with you hair uncovered for 20-30 minutes.

4. Rinse your hair with cool water, then use a gentle, sulfate-free shampoo to wash and proceed with gentle styling. I also recommend the pre-poo process when there is significant scalp scaling in the form or Seborrheic Dermatitis (see Chapter 13) or Psoriasis/Sebopsoriasis (see Chapter 14).

5. For Victoria, after shampooing, I recommended that she towel-dry her hair prior to applying a leave-in conditioner. Just as a dry sponge absorbs more moisture than a wet sponge, your hair will absorb more moisture from your conditioner when it is dry. By eliminating the damaging hair styling practices and making healthy hair care choices, the breakage stopped and Victoria's new hair growth was the healthiest hair she had ever experienced.

TRACTION ALOPECIA
(THIN EDGES)

WHAT IS TRACTION ALOPECIA?

Traction Alopecia (TA), as the name suggests, is hair loss primarily caused by styles that place tension on the hair follicles over long periods of time. As a dermatologist, I have witnessed the fear or helplessness that people immediately feel when they hear the word "alopecia" associated with their particular form of hair loss. The good news is this type of hair loss is completely preventable.

TA occurs when the hair follicles are placed under tension by chronic use of hairstyling practices, including, but not limited to: tight ponytails, braids or cornrows, dreadlocks, certain hair accessories that grip the hair tightly and are worn repeatedly, and even a condition called "trichotillomania" (see Chapter 6 for more on this form of hair loss). Trichotillomania, a condition caused by the repeated pulling the hair out with the hands, can lead to TA. It generally affects the hairline, causing hair loss around the front of the scalp and at the temples. The follicles on the temples are the most delicate on the entire scalp, which is why they are the first to be lost after lengthy stress on them.

Anyone, regardless of gender, ethnicity, or age, can be affected by TA. However, very similar to the condition discussed in Chapter 5, (Trichorrhexis Nodosa, i.e. breakage), TA is experienced among one-third of women of African descent[20] and 18 percent of the young girls (ages 1-15)[21] it affects wear various forms of what are considered to be traumatic hairstyling (including braids, cornrows, weaves, locs, ponytails, and wig use) for a prolonged period of time. It is the second most common cause of hair loss among African American women and it is also common among Hispanic women who wear chronic tight ponytails. Many celebrities, dancers, and models are also greatly affected by this condition due to their frequent use of hair extensions, glued-in and sewn-in hair weaves, hair pieces, etc. Even young children who keep their hair cornrowed or in multiple, small ponytails can get tiny bumps of inflammation along the hairline called, Traction Folliculitis. Traction Folliculitis is often the precursor of TA. Traction Folliculitis can lead to permanent hair loss if not treated and is allowed to progress to scarring.

A PATIENT'S EXPERIENCE WITH TA

Lydia, an early 20-year-old African American female college student, came to my office because the hair around her temples, in

---

20 Khumalo NP, Jessop S, Gumedze F, & Ehrlich R. Hairdressing and the prevalence of scalp disease in African adults. *Br J Dermatol.* 2007;157:981–988.

21 Wright DR, Gathers R, et al. Hair care practices and their association with scalp and hair disorders in African American girls. *J Am Acad Dermatol.* 2011;64:253–262.

front of her ears, and the hairline along her forehead had become alarmingly thin. Her hair was styled into 14 intricate cornrows and pulled tightly at the back with a pony tail holder. In my practice, I often see patients with TA who have worn their hair for months or years in tight braids, corn rows, dreadlocks, sister locs, traditional locs, pony tails or pigtails, or added hair extensions or weaves. Lydia had begun wearing braids in high school, and had not worn her hair natural since the 9th grade when she had her hair locked. Since then, she had worn glued-in weaves twice, followed by six months of braids. She was enjoying the low maintenance of the current cornrow braids that her stylist washed and replaced every two months. Unfortunately, this hairstyle more than likely exacerbated her condition. Lydia also mentioned to me that her two younger sisters, one in middle school and one in high school, are starting to experience peer pressure to chemically relax their hair and to wear long weaves. This peer pressure to chemically relax the hair and wear weaves is something that many teenage African American women experience. As a result of this, is more common among women who wear traction hairstyles on chemically relaxed hair. I call this the "deadly duo". Research out of South Africa found the highest risk of TA occurred when braids were done on relaxed hair.[22] Braids or weaves should never be added to relaxed hair. I encouraged Lydia to share this information with her little sisters.

I performed a thorough scalp examination on Lydia to check for signs of scarring or inflammation, characteristics that are common amongst those who suffer from TA. Not surprisingly, her hairline was slightly tender to touch. The years of tension on her hair follicles had caused some inflammation as evidenced by the redness

---

22 Khumalo NP, Jessop S, et al. Hairdressing is associated with scalp disease in African schoolchil-dren. *Br J Dermatol.* 2007 Jul;157(1):106–110.

that I could see on trichoscopy (see Fig. 6A). A few small pus-filled bumps called pustules were visible at her temples as well. Fortunately for Lydia, she was seeking treatment early enough before the inflammation had done permanent damage and scarring to her hair follicles as I could see tiny hairs called vellus hairs present. Her hair loss pattern was positive for the "fringe sign," which is a small fringe of hairs along the hairline.

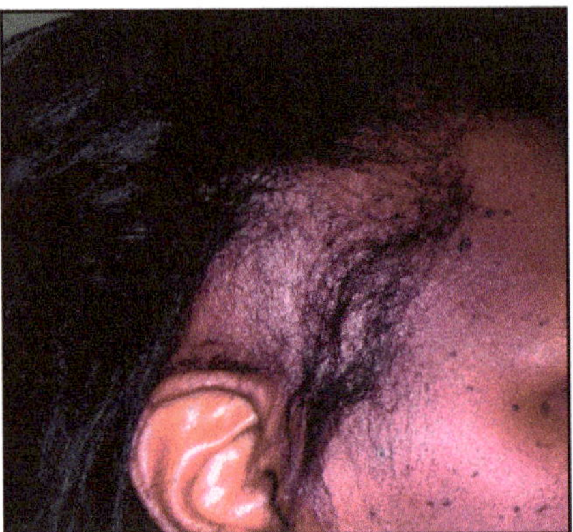

Figure 6A) Traction Alopecia with the Fringe Sign

Lydia's hair also had thinning in a horseshoe pattern at the crown where prior glued-in weaves had been placed. I recommended that hair weaves be left in for shorter periods of time (no longer than four to six weeks) and the minimal possible amount of hair should be used to minimize added weight causing traction on the hair follicles where it attaches to the scalp.

TREATMENT OF TA

After explaining to Lydia the causes for her condition, it made sense to her that the most important part of her treatment plan would be to discontinue any offending traumatic hair styling practices and take what I like to call, a "braid-and-weave holiday," or a break from any hair styling practices that place added tension or weight on the follicles. I recommend this for all of my patients as a preventative measure for further damage. Don't get me wrong, I enjoy braids as a beautiful art form and a wonderful expression of creativity, but an important principle to remember is that your hairstyle should never cause you pain. PAIN EQUALS DAMAGE! When wearing braids, it is important to make sure you can turn your head from side to side after each braid is installed without pain. If it hurts, it is important to request the braider to un-do and re-install the braid until it is comfortable. Pain means damage is occurring to the hair follicle and that damage can lead to permanent scarring and hair loss. I recommend that patients do not leave styles in that create tension on the follicles for no longer than three to four weeks. After that time, I recommend taking them out to give the follicles a rest. I recommend the follicles have at least two to three months of rest in between traction hair styles.

Because Lydia had some visible inflammation at her temples, I prescribed a topical steroid ointment, her preferred formulation, for the affected areas three times weekly. I also gave her a series of injections of an anti-inflammatory steroid into the thinning areas, six to eight weeks apart. My recommendations also included a choice of daily application of Minoxidil 5% foam or a dietary supplement containing marine proteins or saw palmetto as the active ingredient (see Chapter 19 for more information on nutrition and hair and dietary supplements) to thicken the residual hairs along the hairline. Lydia also decided to give her hair a break by wearing a short, natural TWA (Teenie Weenie Afro) just as Victoria (discussed in Chapter 5) did. This allowed her to keep her scalp healthy, clean, and moisturized during the months of treatment. At her six-month visit, Lydia had experienced significant regrowth. Many cases of TA improve six to nine months after discontinuing the offending hairstyling practices. Because TA is a "biphasic" form of hair loss, meaning that it is initially non-scarring, the follicles are still healthy and capable of regrowth.[23] Overtime, with continued use of the causative hair styles, permanent damage of the follicles can occur, preventing the possibility of growth. Hence, early detection and treatment are key!

A NOTE ABOUT HAIR AND PHYSICAL HEALTH

One of Lydia's concerns was not being able to resort to her go-to styles of cornrows, braids, etc., when she participated in intense aerobics classes. In the past, her cornrows allowed her the freedom to exercise without having to frequently redo her hair. This is a frequent concern of African American women seeking to increase physical activity. In a study out of Wake Forest University (among 103 women), one-third of African American women cited the number one reason for not engaging in as much exercise as they would like was because of their hair.[24] The former Surgeon General, Dr. Regina Benjamin, spoke out on the issue as a "public health crisis." She encouraged the nation not to choose "hair over health." Eighty percent of African American women are overweight or obese.[17] Since hair can be a barrier to exercising, Dr. Benjamin joined forces with the Bronner Brothers Hair Show and United Healthcare's "Hair Fitness Initiative," to challenge stylists to create fashionable, exercise-friendly hairstyles to help African American women lead healthy, active lives. There are many exercise-friendly styles that can help facilitate staying active and beautiful. Great options include: twist outs, bantu knots, rocking

---

23 Billero V, Miteva M. Traction alopecia: The root of the problem. *Clin Cosmet Investig Dermatol.* 2018 Apr 6;11:149–159.

24 Hall RR, Francis S, et al. Hair care practices as a barrier to physical activity in African American women. *JAMA Dermatol.* 2013;Mar;149(3):310–14.

a TWA (AKA a teenie weenie afro), a permrod or flexi-rod set or a loose bun. Incorporating hair care aids to use while exercising like the Gymwrap made out of EvapoTech™, a patented material that minimizes sweat absorption through a blend of fabrics, which allows heat to escape while letting cool air in can help preserve while exercising. We should not have to choose between our bodies and our hair. It requires creativity and collaboration with a skilled hair stylist. I always say what value is a beautiful hairstyle if you are hospitalized or bed-ridden because of serious illnesses, many of which regular moderate-intensity physical activity has been shown to help prevent. Researchers looking at data from nearly a half-million people found that high fitness levels decreased the risk of coronary heart disease by 49% and abnormal heart rhythms called arrhythmias by 60% even among those genetically at risk.[25]

Choose wisely...HEALTH OVER HAIR!

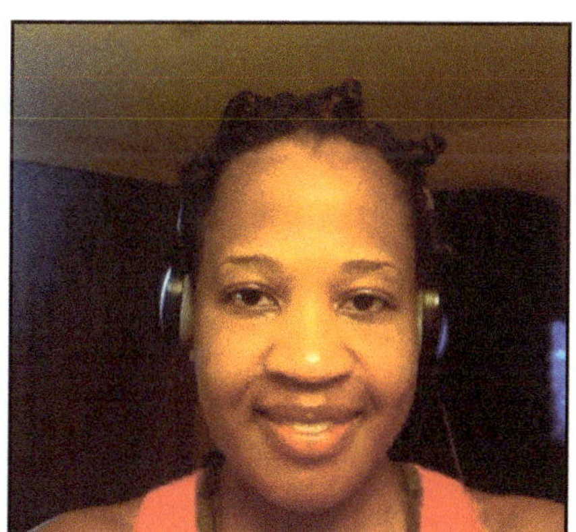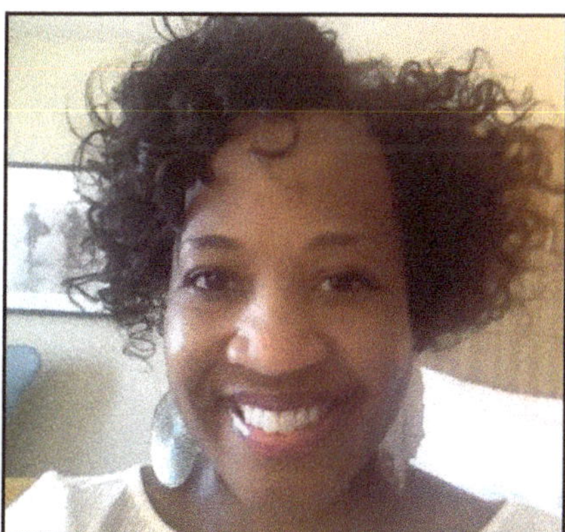

Figure 6B) Bantu Knots are an easy way to transition from working out to getting ready for work!

---

25 Tikkanen E, Gustafsson S, Ingelsson E. Associations of Fitness, Physical Activity, Strength, and Genetic Risk with Cardiovascular Disease: Longitudinal Analyses in the UK Biobank Study. *Circulation*. 2018 Jun 12;137(24):2583-2591.

TINEA CAPITIS
(RINGWORM)

WHAT IS TINEA CAPITIS?

Tinea Capitis (TC) is the clinical name for what is commonly referred to as ringworm or fungal infection of the scalp. TC most commonly occurs in children between 3 and 14 years of age and is the second to Alopecia Areata (AA) in being the most common cause of hair loss seen in children. TC happens when a fungus called a dermatophyte infects the hair and scalp. In the United States, the most prevalent species or type of fungus causing TC is called *Trichophyton tonsurans,* while *Microsporum canus* is the most common form in Europe. It is important to know the species or specific type of fungus causing TC, as the species determines the specific treatment used. For reasons unknown, TC is more common among children of African descent. TC is highly contagious and organisms have been cultured from combs, caps, pillowcases, toys, and theater seats.[26] Studies have found that even after shedding, hairs may harbor fungus for more than one year.[27] While the use of hair grease or oils can increase the risk of dandruff (see Seborrheic Dermatitis, Chapter 13), a similar increase was not found in TC. In a study examining the role of hair care practices in the development of TC, hairstyling, frequency of washing, use of oils or grease, and other hair care practices were not shown to be associated with the presence of TC.[28]

A PATIENT'S EXPERIENCE WITH TC

Jayson, a four-year-old African American male, was referred to my office by his pediatrician for evaluation of two extremely itchy patches of hair loss on the central scalp (Fig. 7A). His mom was told that the daycare would not allow him back in without a doctor's note. I examined Jayson's scalp and saw two large, scaly patches of hair loss. After examining his scalp, I felt enlarged lymph nodes in his neck, which is a common finding in TC. I performed a swab culture of the scaly patches to confirm the presence of fungus and the specific species present. His mom stated that he recently completed a four-week course of Griseofulvin, the oral anti-fungal his pediatrician prescribed without much improvement. Because my clinical suspicion was high that he had resistant TC, I started him on the Ultramicronized Griseofulvin for eight weeks and scheduled him for a follow-up exam to re-culture his

---

26 Schieke SS and Garg A. (2012). Superficial Fungal Infection. In Fitzpatrick's Dermatology in General Medicine (p. 2285). McGraw-Hill.

27 Howard R, Frieden IJ: Tinea capitis: New perspectives on an old disease. *Semin Dermatol.* 1995 Mar;14(1):2-8.

28 Sharma V, Silverberg NB, et al. Do hair care practices affect the acquisition of tinea capitis? A case-control study. *Arch Pediatr Adolesc Med.* 2001;Jul;155(7):818–21.

scalp at that time. Four weeks later the culture results were positive for *Trichophyton tonsurans*. During his second follow-up visit, there was significant improvement in the scaling and signs of mild hair re-growth. I re-cultured the scalp. After four weeks, the culture results were negative and the lymph nodes in his neck had gone down.

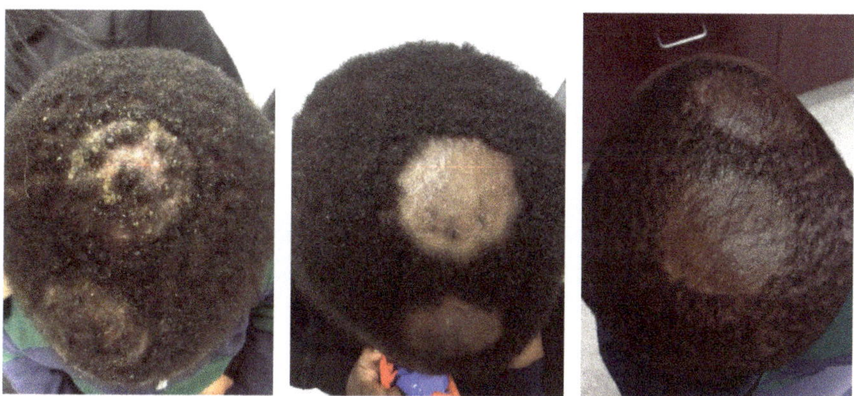

Figure 7A) – Tinea Capitis Before Treatment – After 3 weeks Oral Antifungal – After 6 weeks Oral Antifungal

TREATMENT FOR TC

One of the common misconceptions regarding the treatment of TC is that medicated shampoos can adequately treat it. Because the fungal infection is located within the hair follicle, which emanates from beneath the scalp, treatment must be systemic through the bloodstream. The gold standard treatment for TC is oral griseofuvin, which comes in two forms: griseofulvin microsize 20-25 mg/kg/day and griseofulvin ultramicrosize 15 mg/kg/day taken in divided doses with a fatty meal for 8 weeks. It is recommended to take griseofulvin with a fatty meal as it has been found to increase absorption. The current recommendations are not evidenced-based on controlled trials, but are based on collective clinical experience suggesting high therapeutic effectiveness. Terbinafine is an alternative, which is also FDA approved for TC in a granular formulation sprinkled on food for six weeks. In a recent analysis comparing treatments for tinea capitis, for infections caused by Microsporum species, griseofulvin was superior (p = 0.04), whereas terbinafine was superior for infections caused by Trichophyton species infection (p = 0.04).[29] In addition to the systemic oral medication, I also prescribed an antifungal shampoo like Ketoconazole 2% or Ciclopirox shampoo to reduce the contagious nature of TC both in the patient as well as with household contacts.

---

29 Gupta AK1, Drummond-Main C. Meta-analysis of randomized, controlled trials comparing partic-ular doses of griseofulvin and terbinafine for the treatment of tinea capitis. Pediatr Dermatol. 2013 Jan-Feb;30(1):1-6.

TRICHOTILLOMANIA
(HAIR PULLING)

WHAT IS TRICHOTILLOMANIA?

Trichotillomania (TTM) is a psycho-dermatologic disorder first described in 1889 by Francois Henri Hallopeau, as an uncontrollable urge to pull one's own hair. It is usually associated with depression and obsessive compulsive disorder and for this reason, it is considered an anxiety disorder. The onset of TTM varies from 9-13 years of age and is more common in females. It only affects about one percent of the adult population but can occur at any age. Some patients with this disorder tend to pull large amounts of hair out, causing irregularly-shaped patches of hair loss at the site. The scalp, eyebrows, and eyelashes are the most commonly affected sites of TTM; however, any body area may be affected by this disorder. Many who suffer from TTM ingest the hair after pulling it, causing gastrointestinal problems as well. Although it is a psychiatric condition, many patients with the disorder first see a dermatologist. Alopecia Areata (AA) is another condition that shares similar signs or symptoms and because of this, some TTM patients are initially diagnosed with AA before being diagnosed with TTM. As mentioned in Chapter 4, AA is the most common form of hair loss found in children.

Some of the possible causes of TTM include situations that may trigger the children emotionally. TTM can happen as a result of a child experiencing separation from an attachment figure, birth of a younger sibling or sibling rivalry, moving into a new house, or even problems with school performance. It is believed that environment is a factor as well because the hair pulling behavior usually takes place when children are alone and in a relaxed environment. Unfortunately, due to the aesthetic results of TTM, it can have a negative impact on a patient's quality of life. A patient can become withdrawn socially, personally, and in the case of adults, occupationally.

Diagnosis of TTM has remained challenging for clinicians today because of the commonalities it has with AA, which can lead to a misdiagnosis. Patients with TTM show signs of "bizarre-shaped," irregular alopecia patches formed by multiple broken hairs. Many patients who suffer from this condition hide the fact that they pull their hair from their family and friends, which contributes to the difficulty of diagnosing TTM. In light of the diagnosis challenge, trichoscopy (the examination of the scalp using a trichoscope) has emerged as a noninvasive and useful tool in the diagnosis of both TTM and AA (Fig. 8A and Fig. 8B). This method has been proven to increase diagnostic accuracy and reduce the need for biopsy. Some common characteristics of a TTM diagnosis include: black dots, coiled hairs, tulip hairs, and hook hairs, to name a few. Exclamation point hairs, which are suggestive of AA, are usually absent.

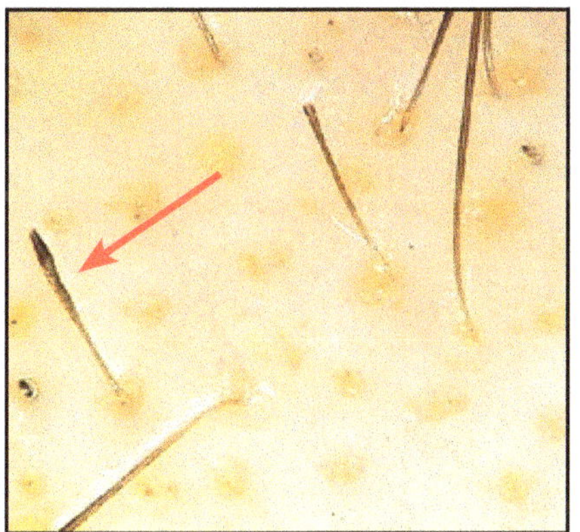

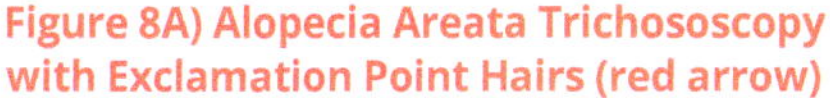

Figure 8A) Alopecia Areata Trichososcopy with Exclamation Point Hairs (red arrow)

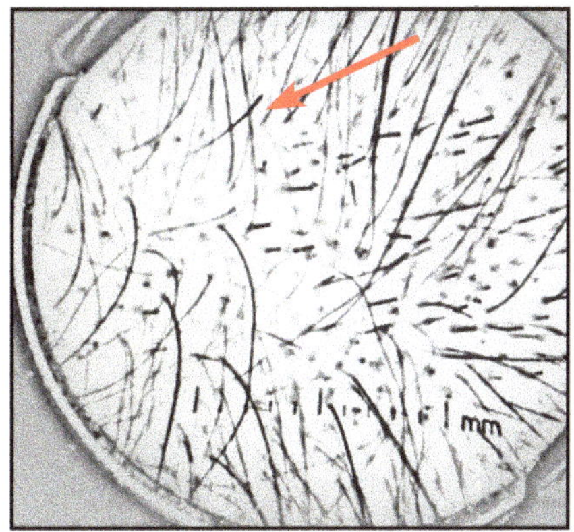

Figure 8B) Trichotillomania Trichoscopy with Fractured Ends (red arrow)

A PATIENT'S EXPERIENCE WITH TRICHOTILLOMANIA

Meaghan, a 12-year-old Caucasian female, came to my office with her mother because her mom noticed a large patch of hair loss behind her daughter's right ear, as well as patches in her eyelashes and eyebrows for the past six weeks. Naturally she was concerned. After speaking with the patient and her mom, the mother revealed that her daughter had become withdrawn since she recently separated from her father. This revelation was followed by the little girl admitting that, at night and in bed, she would often find herself "twisting and twirling" her hair.

I examined Meaghan's scalp and saw a large, lancet-shaped patch of hair loss with a tuft of remaining hairs in the center of the patch on the right nape of the scalp (Fig. 8C). There were also small patches of hair loss on the eyebrows, which on dermoscopy revealed that the follicles were still open, consistent with a non-scarring hair loss. I performed a "pull test" around the border of the patch of hair loss on the scalp, in which I gently tugged on about 25 hairs from the root to the end, which resulted in only one–two hairs coming out, which is considered a normal pull test.

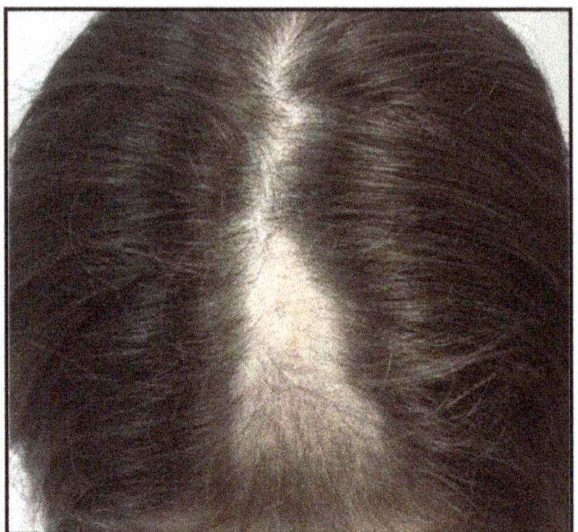

Figure 8C) Trichotillomania

After performing the examination, I recommended that we perform a scalp biopsy to confirm my strong suspicion of TTM. For diagnoses like TTM a biopsy is often helpful for providing a definitive diagnosis given there is sometimes denial of the pulling behavior.

Meaghan's biopsy returned with pigmented hair casts and trichomalacia (or deformed hair shafts) consistent with TTM. Therefore, I recommended she see a local child psychologist who specializes in helping children with anxiety and life transitions. Her mom was relieved to know that the condition was not life-threatening and often could be treated with various strategies of therapy alone or in combination with an anti-depressant.

TREATMENT FOR TTM

Unfortunately, the research on treatment for TTM is very limited. A wide variety of treatments have been used to treat symptoms in children, adolescents, and adults. Behavioral therapy for the condition still lacks scientific evidence and all findings are based on case reports. However, some treatment options have helped patients either reduce the pulling of their hair or stop all together. In addition to therapy, there are certain medications that have also proven to be effective in the treatment of TTM.

Behavioral Therapy

Habit reversal training – One method that has proven effective for TTM is habit reversal training. When this method is applied, you are instructed to first recognize situations that may cause you to engage in hair pulling. When you notice that you are engaging in pulling, you are to consciously substitute other behaviors instead to redirect. For example, instead of placing your hand in the hair, you would redirect your hand to your ear, or instead of pulling on your hair, you would simply clench your fists.

Cognitive therapy – This form of therapy helps to identify and evaluate any negative beliefs that they may have linked to your hair pulling.

Medications

Currently, the FDA has not approved any medications for the treatment of TTM. However, there are certain drugs that have proven helpful in case reports and case series. Drugs such as lithium, tricyclic antidepressants, selective serotonin reuptake inhibitors

(SSRIs), and antipsychotics have been found to be successful with controlling certain symptoms. An alternative offered for SSRIs, due to their high dosage side effects include glutamate modulating agents such as N-acetylcysteine, which acts by reducing oxidative stress. It is widely used and does not require a prescription. In some cases of TTM, which occurred due to sibling rivalry, treatment consisted of a combination of cognitive behavioral therapy (such as the ones mentioned above), mild topical steroids, mild shampoo, and methionine (an amino acid containing sulfur). With parental help and cooperation, patients showed significant improvement.

Although the most common time of onset of TTM is during childhood, there are surprisingly very few TTM research studies that include adolescents or children. The initial findings for behavioral therapy have been very encouraging, however. This still leaves a big question mark pertaining to the role of developmental factors in TTM development and the response to treatment. In cases where cognitive behavioral therapy was used alone to treat adults, a relapse in behavior proved to be problematic for some. In cases where SSRIs were used, they seemed to have no effect on reducing hair pulling symptoms.[30] There have been a few randomized controlled trials in which combined treatments of medication plus behavioral therapy have been successful.[31] However, there have not been many studies of the two combined treatments. It can be said for sure however, that for children diagnosed with TTM, a collaborative effort between the parents, patients and physicians are key for successful management.

---

30 Franklin ME, Zagrabbe K, Benavides KL. Trichotillomania and its treatment: A review and rec-ommendations. *Expert Rev Neurother.* 2011 Aug;11(8):1165–74.

31 Pinto AC, Andrade TC, et al. Trichotillomania: A case report with clinical differential diagnosis and dermatoscopic with alopecia areata. *An Bras Dermatol.* 2017;92(1):118–20.

ANAGEN EFFLUVIUM
(CHEMOTHERAPY HAIR LOSS)

WHAT IS ANAGEN EFFLUVIUM?

As discussed in earlier chapters, anagen, catagen, and telogen are the three major phases of the human hair growth cycle. Anagen is the "growing" phase, catagen is the "transitional" phase, and telogen is the "resting" phase. Anagen effluvium (AE) is the abrupt loss of hairs that are in their growing phase due to an event that impairs the metabolic activity of hair follicle. It is commonly observed as a result of radiotherapy to the head and neck or chemotherapeutic agents. Whether or not one experiences hair loss from chemotherapy depends mostly on the type and dose of medication prescribed. These agents can impair or totally disrupt the anagen cycle and cause varying degrees of hair loss. Since 80 percent to 90 percent of scalp hairs are in the anagen phase, a large number of hairs are affected. It is estimated that 65 percent of patients taking chemotherapy will experience hair loss.

Unfortunately, many of us know someone who has experienced the awful monster known as cancer. Both men and women report hair loss as one of the side effects they fear most after being diagnosed with cancer. During the growth phase of the hair cycle, there is an injury of the keratinocytes (the epidermal cells that produce keratin) in the hair matrix, which causes the hair that grows out of the scalp to become weakened with the slightest manipulation, which leads to breakage in the anagen phase and results in the hair falling out. In other words, the chemotherapy and radiation creates a toxic breeding ground for the hair follicles, making them unable to grow because the damage is basically occurring at the root. Because of this, it is often referred to as "toxic alopecia." It's quite similar to attempting to grow plants in toxic soil. When the hair is suffering from AE, hair loss can begin within one to two weeks of starting chemotherapy and patients can lose more than 80 percent to 90 percent of scalp hair with two to three months.[32] The hair loss often starts from the crown and sides of the scalp, which could be due to the increased friction during sleep and wearing head coverings. Chemotherapy given at high doses for a long duration may also affect hairs of the beard, eyebrows, and eyelashes, as well as the armpits and pubic regions. Most patients will have regrowth within one to three months after stopping chemotherapy. In 60 percent of the cases, this regrowth can be a different texture or color. It might be curlier than it was before, or it could be gray until the cells that control the pigment in hair begin to function again.

Chemotherapy-induced hair loss has a great impact on the quality of a patient's life. It has a negative impact on an individual's perception of appearance, body image, sexuality, and self-esteem.

---

32 Sellheyer K, Bergfeld WF. Non-Neoplastic Disorders of Hair. In *Dermatopathology*, 2010.

In a study, 47 percent of female patients considered hair loss to be the most traumatic aspect of chemotherapy, and 8 percent declined chemotherapy due to fears of hair loss.[33]

A PATIENT'S EXPERIENCE WITH AE: MRS. BEULAH WHITE

There is one thing that doctors tell chemo patients, "With certainty, you will lose your hair." Studies show that women with cancer consider hair loss due to chemotherapy the most devastating aspect. It does not stop most of them because only 8 percent say they would refuse chemo for that very reason. There is a third group not included in the study. These are the women who place greater emphasis on healing than having a head of hair.

In the winter of 2017, I was diagnosed with Triple Negative, Stage III breast cancer that had progressed to my lymph nodes in my arm. This means that I would undergo the most aggressive forms of chemotherapy, then surgery, and finally radiation. I knew that this prognosis was grim and I initially did not think about the hair loss.

My dance with hair loss due to chemo was gradual. Dealing with tufts of hair on my pillow or the clumps in the shower was absent-mindedly abnormal. I was having such severe reactions to the chemo that my hair was the last thing on my mind. Life is full of contradictions. Once I began combing out handfuls of hair, it got my attention. I couldn't style it because the texture had changed. I dilly dallied. I would look in the mirror several times during the day imagining my head bald.

---

33 Trüeb RM. Chemotherapy-induced hair loss. *Skin Therapy Lett.* 2010;15:5–7.

After two rounds of chemotherapy or about four weeks in to the treatment plan, I decided to cut my losses. I asked a barber friend of mine to come to my home. Upon arrival, he asked, "How do you want it cut"? I told him to take it all off. No one talked. The only sound was the buzz of the clippers and the soft sound of my hair hitting the floor.

I am progressing through my bout with cancer, I just finished my rounds of radiation on November 17, 2017. My hair is finally starting to grow back. As it is beginning to grow back, my hair's texture seems to have changed. It is coming back in softer and more manageable. As I am writing this, my hair is barely more than a buzz cut, yet I am so grateful to be a cancer survivor! I fully realize that my hair will eventually grow back. As my strength returns, my hair is growing. I view it as a resurgence of my health and vitality, and a tremendous testament to my survival.

TREATMENT FOR AE

While there aren't any treatments that prevent AE from occurring all together, there have been certain treatments/techniques used to decrease the loss of hair once chemotherapy and radiation treatments have stopped and to regenerate hair growth at a faster rate.

Scalp cooling via use of penguin caps – This method of treatment, while not able to prevent hair loss altogether, does aid in reduction. This method works by cooling the scalp causing the blood vessels to constrict, which is believed to limit the amount of the chemo carried to the hair follicles. In a study conducted beginning August 2013 until October 2014, women with Stage I or Stage II breast cancer receiving non-anthracycline-based chemotherapy participated in a study that focused on the effects of using a scalp cooling system 30 minutes prior to their chemotherapy cycles. The scalp temperatures were maintained at 3°C throughout the treatment and for 90 to 120 minutes after the treatment ended. Among the 122 patients in the study, hair loss of less than 50% was found in 67 to 101 patients, four weeks after the end of their chemo treatments.

Minoxidil – Minoxidil is a topical medication applied to the scalp to stimulate hair growth. One of the most popular brands known among the public today is Rogaine. Topical Minoxidil has been shown to shorten the duration of hair loss due to chemotherapy and/or radiation by approximately 50 days, but it is unable to prevent hair loss due to cancer chemotherapy or radiation therapy.[34] It primarily serves to accelerate hair growth after the chemo/radiation treatments have ended.

Patient education is very important in AE as alopecia can be psychologically devastating to a patient. Appropriate hair and scalp care along with temporarily wearing a wig or hair replacement unit may be the most effective coping strategies for these patients.

Recommendations for hair care include:

- Gentle hair care practices (e.g. avoiding bleaching, coloring, perming, or using excessive heat appliances).

- Use a satin pillowcase, which is less likely to attract and catch fragile hair.

---

34 Hood AF. Cutaneous side effects of cancer chemotherapy. *Med Clin North Am.* 1986 Jan;70(1):187–209.

- Use a soft brush and shampooing with a gentle shampoo. Cutting hair shorter as it looks fuller than longer hair, and when the hair is shed, it is less noticeable when the hair has already been short. Moreover, hair that has been cut short may help patients to ease the transition to total alopecia. Many insurance plans provide coverage for a wig or hair replacement system for patients with chemotherapy-induced alopecia.

- Consume food that promotes hair growth and a strong immune system. For more information on the topic of food and hair growth, check out my e-book "Dr. Lenzy's Hair Diet," which is available at www.LenzyDerm.com.

- Finally, support groups are offered throughout the United States and in several other countries, which provide resources to help patients cope not only with the hair loss associated with cancer treatments but other aspects as well.

CENTRAL CENTRIFUGAL CICATRICIAL ALOPECIA
(#1 CAUSE OF HAIR LOSS IN BLACK WOMEN)

WHAT IS CENTRAL CENTRIFUGAL CICATRICIAL ALOPECIA?

CCCA is the acronym for the most common cause of hair loss in African American women. It stands for: **Central** (because it begins at the crown), **Centrifugal** (because it expands or spreads outward over time), **Cicatricial** (which is the Latin word for scarring), and Alopecia (which means hair loss). As we've discussed in previous chapters, hair loss affects all ages, races, and ethnicities, but in African American women, CCCA is the most common cause of hair loss. If it is untreated, the hair loss expands outward from the center of the scalp, and scarring prevents hair re-growth. Once the follicle has been destroyed, no hair will grow back.

There are very few published research studies that indicate how prevalent CCCA is. Two studies of over 200 patients place the occurrence between 2.7% and 5.6% of African American women studied. Based on clinical experience, however, these estimates appear to be low. CCCA can begin in women as early as their twenties, typically beginning before their forties. Because the onset is so gradual, many patients do not realize they need to seek treatment. Unfortunately, those delays often result in more extensive hair loss and irreversible scarring.

While the exact cause of CCCA is not known, there are three possible culprits that may contribute to this form of hair loss: genetics, hair styling practices and chemical relaxers. Published studies suggest that there is a genetic component associated with CCCA because it often runs in families of those diagnosed.[35] Styling that traumatizes the hair follicle (i.e. traction hair styles such as tight braids and weaves) places gentle pressure on the roots over hours or days and can cause an inflammatory reaction in the scalp. This inflammatory reaction in the scalp, can lead to scarring over time. As a matter of fact, these hairstyles were associated with the most severe cases of hair loss at the crown and middle of the scalp.[36] Chemical relaxers were found to be used among 94 percent of the patients diagnosed with CCCA. In a study of 529 African American women, 496 (90%) of the women had used relaxers but there was no association of relaxer use and CCCA.[37]

35　Dlova NC, Jordaan FH, Sarig O, & Sprecher E. Autosomal dominant inheritance of central cen-trifugal cicatricial alopecia in black South Africans. *J Am Acad Dermatol.* 2014;70(4):679–682.

36　Gathers RC, Jankowski M, Eide M, & Lim HW. Hair grooming practices and central centrifugal cicatricial alopecia. *J Am Acad Dermatol.* 2009 Apr;60(4):574–578.

37　Olsen EA, Callender V, McMichael A, Sperling L, Anstrom KJ, Shapiro J, Roberts J, et al. Cen-tral hair loss in African American women: incidence and potential risk factors. *J Am Acad Dermatol.* 2011 Feb;64(2):245–252.

Chemical relaxers can definitely play a role in weakening the hair shaft, which can lead to breakage. However, an interesting discovery in this study was that, while 94% of the women in the group diagnosed with CCCA used chemical relaxers, the women in the control group NOT diagnosed with CCCA had used chemical relaxers as well. Due to the many products and styling practices that women affected with CCCA have used throughout their lives, it is difficult to determine which factors have actually "caused" the hair loss and even more difficult to create a control group of women who have never used such hair grooming practices and products as a whole. This poses some very unique challenges in discovering the cause and determining prevention for CCCA.

A PATIENT'S EXPERIENCE WITH CCCA

Kayla, an African American woman, was referred to my practice by her hair stylist because her hair loss had been gradually expanding over the past four years. She was in excellent health at 43 years of age, which pretty much ruled out any underlying health conditions. During my visit with Kyla at our office, we talked about how long she had noticed her hair thinning and whether her hair loss was from falling out or from breaking off. I asked her about the hair products she used on a regular basis, the styling practices she had used throughout her lifetime, and about her family's experience with hair loss as well. It was evident early on in our conversation that Kayla had meticulously cared for her hair all of her life. As a teen, she began using relaxers and wore tight rows of braids for a month at a time for most of the year. Her hair routine over the last couple of years consisted of sew-in weaves, which helped to hide her thinning crown. She shampooed her hair weekly using a natural olive oil and glycerin shampoo, conditioned her hair using a deep-conditioning treatment, and flat ironed her hair with a ceramic flat iron on a weekly basis. Finally, we talked about any discomfort she had experienced, including itching, burning or tenderness to touch. Although she noticed her scalp was itchy at times, she had not sought any treatment for the problem.

After reviewing Kayla's family history and hair care routine/habits, I moved onto the examination of her hair and scalp. Kayla's hair loss was visible at the top of the scalp in her crown (Fig. 10A). There was evidence of breakage (with hairs of different lengths) throughout her hair upon examination of her scalp using a hair card with a contrasting color as the hair (Fig. 10B). On trichoscopy (Fig. 10C), there was evidence that the hair root, or follicle had scarring, with the loss of the follicle openings. There were multiple white/gray halos, white patches and pinpoint white dots at the hair follicles. When the follicle is scarred, permanent damage occurs, and the follicle cannot be restored. Follicle damage in the form of scarring is central to the diagnosis of CCCA.

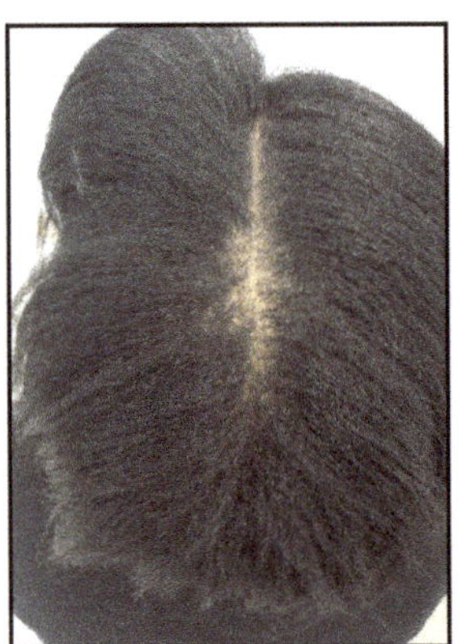

Figure 10A) Early CCCA

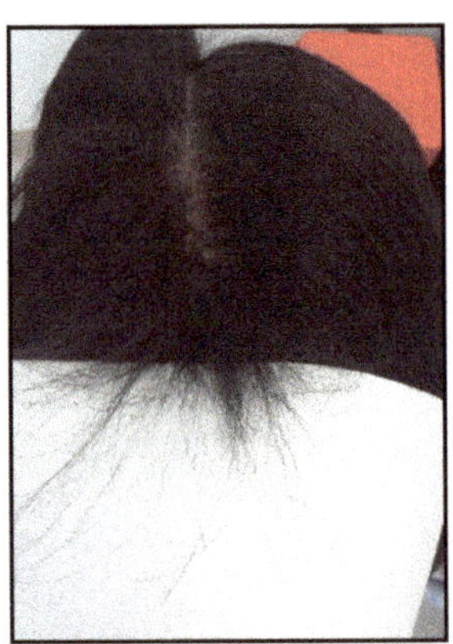

Figure 10B) Breakage in Early CCCA

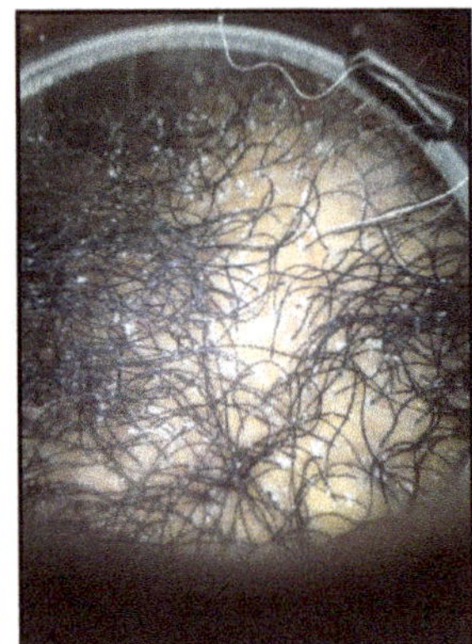

Figure 10C) Trichoscopy of Early CCCA

Very early cases of CCCA are difficult to distinguish from AA so a scalp biopsy can be necessary to make a definitive diagnosis. Sometimes the hair loss progresses to the stage where there are clear signs of follicle destruction and I am able to make the diagnosis without a biopsy; however, wasn't Kayla's case just yet. We took a small biopsy of Kayla's scalp to confirm the diagnosis. Findings such as inflammation, scarring and loss of follicles can be present below the skin and a biopsy gives a clear picture of what is happening at the microscopic level. Kayla's biopsy results returned one week later, showing damage to the sebaceous glands, which are the oil glands below the surface of the scalp, as well as scarring and inflammation around the follicles. This confirmed to me that Kayla was definitely experiencing CCCA.

TREATMENT OF CCCA

Kayla had previously heard of CCCA because her mother had experienced hair loss. I explained to her that the goal of treatment is to relieve her symptoms of itching and tenderness and prevent progression of follicle destruction and scarring. We talked about using a topical steroid (which comes in several formulations, including an ointment that has the consistency of Vaseline, cream, foam, or solution), using steroid injections at the sites of inflammation, and taking an anti-inflammatory medication. Injections along the edge of the hair loss area can help to prevent the expansion of the affected area. Kayla decided to use the topical steroid ointment and consider the steroid injections at her two-month follow-up appointment only if there was any sign of further progression of her symptoms.

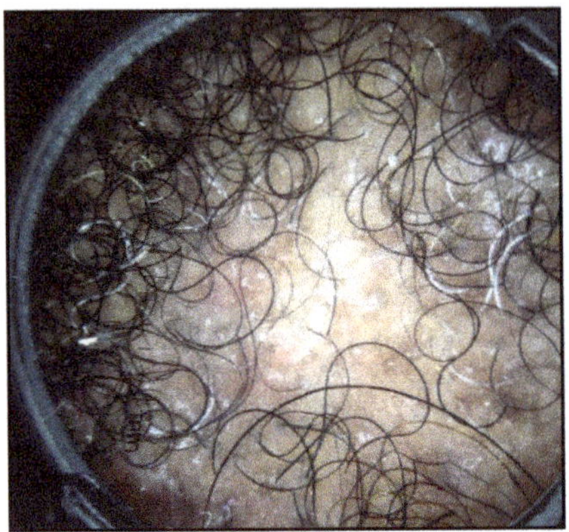

Figure 10D) Trichoscopy of Late Stage CCCA

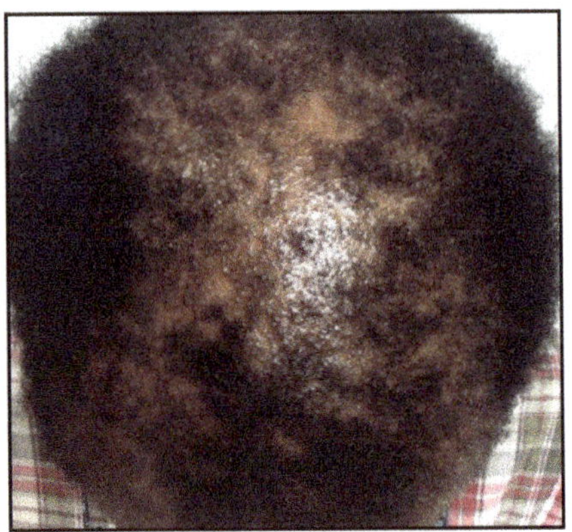

Figure 10E) Late Stage CCCA Before Treatment

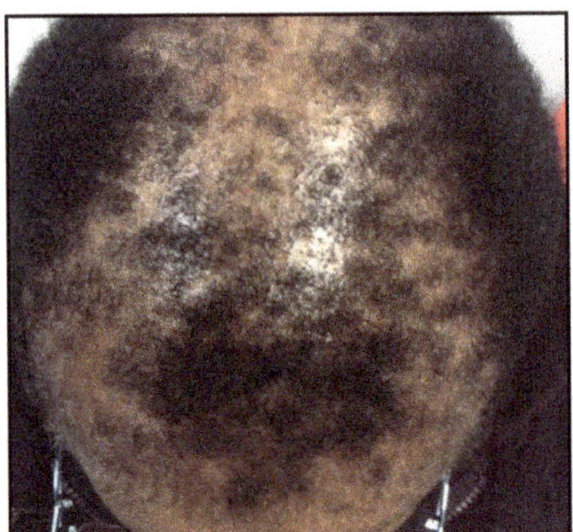

Figure 10E) Late Stage CCCA After 2 months of Topical Clobetasol 3x/week only (Worsening)

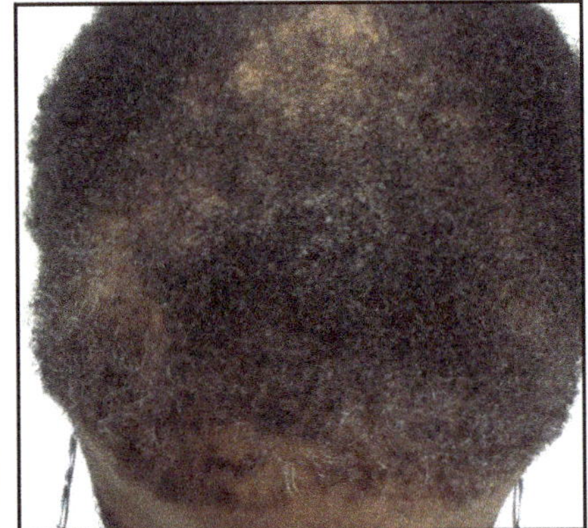

Figure 10F) Late Stage CCCA After 7 Months of Treatment: 3 Monthly Triamcinolone Injections Topical Clobetasol 3x/week Minoxidil 5% Foam Daily

Once CCCA is stabilized, a maintenance regimen could include adding a hair growth aid to help thickening the remaining hairs and provide coverage for the area of hair loss like Minoxidil 5% foam to increase the size of the often miniaturized or small hair follicles often co-existent in women with CCCA. I also often recommend supplements with clinical trial evidence like Viviscal Professional (with active ingredients including marine proteins) and Nutrafol (with active ingredients including saw palmetto, curcumin and Ashwaganda root) to help thicken the remaining hairs by reversing the miniaturization. A safe hair care recommendation list is also an essential part of the treatment plan. I use these recommendations as guidelines to protect your hair health while the treatments described above address the inflammation to prevent further scarring as well as any coexistent miniaturization of the follicles:

- If possible, choose a natural hair style.

- If you choose to stay relaxed:
    - Use mild strength relaxers.
    - Stretch frequency of use from every 6-8 weeks to every 10-12 weeks.

- Limit heat (blow dryers, hot combs, and flat irons) to once a week to freshly shampooed hair.

- Minimize traction (weave/braids).

- Have weave/braid holidays greater than or equal to the length of time the style was installed.

- Don't ignore scalp symptoms: itching, tenderness, or pain. As mentioned in the previous chapter on Traction Alopecia, pain means damage!

When CCCA is diagnosed early, the expansion of scarring can be stopped and steps can be taken to restore the hair to optimal health. Just as with any diagnosis, early detection and treatment are key!

"KEEP ON MOVING"

Virginia D. Miller
(Patient with CCCA)

At 78 years of age, I've experienced a lot in my life – most good, some bad – but through it all, God has kept me. An avid church attendee most of my adult life, there was a brief time in my life where going to my favorite church events caused me slight anxiety and fear. About five years ago, I started noticing my hair was rapidly thinning around the sides and the crown of my head. Initially, I thought it might be a side effect of some new medicine I was taking but when I ceased taking the medicine, the hair loss continued. To cover up my thinning sides I used hair wax and hair gel to slick the longer hairs over my thinning areas – giving the illusion of a full head of hair. This method allowed me to cover things up for a while but within a few months, my thinning led to some bald areas or areas where my hair was no longer than a man's shadow beard. I felt some discouragement because my typical attempts to keep my hair looking normal were no longer effective.

I started using a hairpiece with an elastic band to ensure my head stayed covered. It was even more damaging to my hair. Even though the elastic band was not supposed to cause further damage, every time I took the hairpiece off, my hair – the small amount I had left – would come off with it. But what choice did I have? It was either wear the hairpiece or go uncovered — and I was not ready for the alternative. That's when I saw a commercial for Rogaine and decided to give it a try. I had some brief re-growth but it fell out just as quickly as it came in. I also tried a shampoo for thinning hair with the same results as the Rogaine – regrowth with it all falling back out within a few months. Nothing I was trying was yielding me the results I desired…a normal, full head of hair.

Looking back, I remember the feeling of defeat and some shame. All these years, I'd had a full head of hair, now it was over 60% gone. Getting ready for church became a chore when before it was the highlight of my week. I was not just involved on Sundays but I had choir practice on Tuesdays and bible study on Wednesdays. I did my best to stay positive but was often overcome by my emotions and would leave the house feeling insecure. Would my hairpiece stay in place? I barely had enough hair in the back for the rubber band to hang on to and was afraid that one sudden move would result in my hairpiece falling off or moving to a position where others would see my balding scalp. I went through these emotions for a few weeks and then I decided enough was enough. I wasn't going to live that way anymore. I loved going to church. I loved the life I was living, and I wasn't going to let hair loss steal my joy anymore.

Five years after I noticed my hair thinning I was sitting down at the medical center I attend and noticed a flier for Dr. Lenzy regarding hair loss and alopecia. I took down the information and shared it with one of my daughters. Later that week she was at the hairdresser and discussed my hair loss with her stylist. Her stylist suggested I set up a consultation with one of her other clients – Dr. Lenzy. She told my daughter that Dr. Lenzy was a dermatologist who specialized in hair loss. It felt like a sign for her name to come up twice in just a few weeks, so I made an appointment and had my daughter go with me.

My consultation was very informative and answered a lot of unanswered questions and curiosities I had. I was convinced my hair loss was a result of years of hair perms and over processing. I told Dr. Lenzy the story of going to a salon in a women's home. She would put my perm in and sometimes run out to the store or finish cooking supper, leaving my scalp burning for relief. I would have massive scabs and sores in my head, but every six to eight weeks, I returned. The last perm I got was about eight years ago and it is one I will never forget. The woman perming my hair applied the perm and decided to run out. By the time she returned my scalp was so damaged from the perm that I had puss and extreme tenderness for weeks. I'd finally come to my breaking point. I pledged that after my scalp healed I would never get a perm again. I kept my promise. After sharing my story, while quite concerned, Dr. Lenzy let me know that my hair loss was not a direct correlation with the perms I had received for years.

We went through my family history and although I didn't ever recall hearing the word alopecia, my mom had experienced similar hair loss just as I was experiencing now. In February 2015, I received my diagnosis CCCA. The diagnosis did not come as a shock, and I was happy to finally have a name for my hair loss along with tons of information. Dr. Lenzy gave me her treatment recommendations and we began them right away. I used a steroid cream, which was very effective causing more re-growth than I'd ever experienced during my five-year journey. The re-growth continued for six months, however, it eventually fell out again. I'm still very hopeful that the next treatment will bring sustained re-growth. But even if that is not case, I'm more than okay with me as I am.

As I mentioned earlier, it took some time to get to this place but I realize that despite this one area of my life, I live a good life. I'm 78 years old and still extremely active. I spend three days a week helping other elderly women – ages 83 and 86 – to get around in the community. Since I am still able to drive, I take them to all of their doctor's appointments to pick up meds and to go grocery shopping. I also have a 65-year-old lady I assist who is wheelchair bound. I ride the bus with her whenever she needs to go to the doctor. I thank God for my health. When I stopped focusing on what was lacking in my life and started focusing on all I had, I realized that I had to keep on moving no matter the storms of life.

When my battle with CCCA started five years ago, I was shy and guarded about my situation. Now I take every opportunity to tell others about it, so that they, too, can receive treatment sooner. One of my biggest regrets is not meeting Dr. Lenzy five years earlier. I know if I would have received treatment sooner, I would have better results and less hair loss. So, since I can't change the past, I try to educate others so they can have a better future.

Recently, I was at my niece's graduation and I saw someone who was showing the signs of alopecia. I recognized the discomfort and anxiety in her eyes because I had experienced it myself. When presented the opportunity, I walked with her to the restroom and removed my hairpiece so she could see my scalp. I wanted her to know she wasn't alone but more importantly that she should get help immediately. I was thankful for the chance to help and the courage to stand in my truth without any anxiety or fear. Once fear had me stuck and feeling defeated but now whenever it tries to come around, it's just a reminder to keep on moving.

LICHEN PLANOPILARIS AND FRONTAL FIBROSING ALOPECIA
(HAIR LOSS)

WHAT ARE LICHEN PLANOPILARIS AND FRONTAL FIBROSING ALOPECIA?

Lichen Planopilaris (LPP) is a permanent scarring alopecia that presents itself in one of three types: 1) Classic LPP: Sometimes appears with patches of hair loss throughout the scalp with redness and scaling around the follicles called per-follicular erythema, and scaling, which are signs that the condition is still "active" vs "burnt out." 2) Frontal Fibrosing Alopecia: Clinically similar to LPP, but the hair loss is isolated to the frontal hairline, and can and extend to the sideburns. 3) Graham-Little Syndrome: A very rare condition characterized by LPP of the scalp, and non-scarring hair loss affecting the eyebrows, armpits, groin; and a bumpy rash on other parts of the body.

About 40 percent of scarring alopecia cases seen in my office are caused by LPP. LPP usually appears in middle-aged adults, and is twice as common in women as in men. It is the most frequent cause of scarring alopecia in Caucasian women. The disease starts with redness and scaling around the hair follicles, and because of the scarring to the hair follicles over months or years, it leaves areas of permanent hair loss on the affected areas of the scalp. LPP is the scalp version of an inflammatory skin disease called Lichen Planus. Seventeen to 28 percent of those diagnosed with LPP have symptoms of lichen planus elsewhere on their body. Although the exact cause is unknown, it is believed to be an autoimmune condition.

Frontal Fibrosing Alopecia (FFA) is often seen in post-menopausal women, and for this reason, it has been hypothesized that there is a hormonal component to its cause. Its exact cause is still unknown, but it is the subject of many active studies worldwide. A 2012 study found that 30 percent of patients who have been diagnosed with FFA also have another autoimmune disease. Recent discoveries out of The Cleveland Clinic reveal that LPP may develop as the result of disruption of lipid metabolism in the scalp.

A PATIENT'S EXPERIENCE WITH FFA

Susan, a 50-year-old Caucasian woman, came to my office because of itching, tenderness, and burning on her scalp along her forehead. She had lost hair in a symmetrical pattern across her frontal hairline, and her eyebrows were very sparse. Susan had noticed the hair loss for several months, but the itching had recently increased, causing her to seek treatment. I suspected that Susan was suffering from FFA due to the gradual hair loss and scarring along the frontal hairline and the eyebrows. About 70 percent of those with

FFA also experience eyebrow loss. This is sometimes referred to as the "lonely hair sign" and is indicative of FFA (Fig. 11A). FFA can also occasionally be seen in men as the loss of hair along the frontal hairline or sometimes as isolated sideburn loss (Fig, 11B).

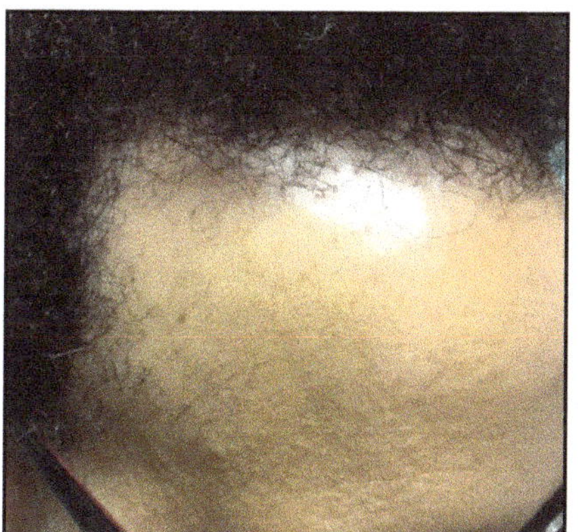

Figure 11A) Example of FFA - "Lonely Hair Sign" & Facial Papules

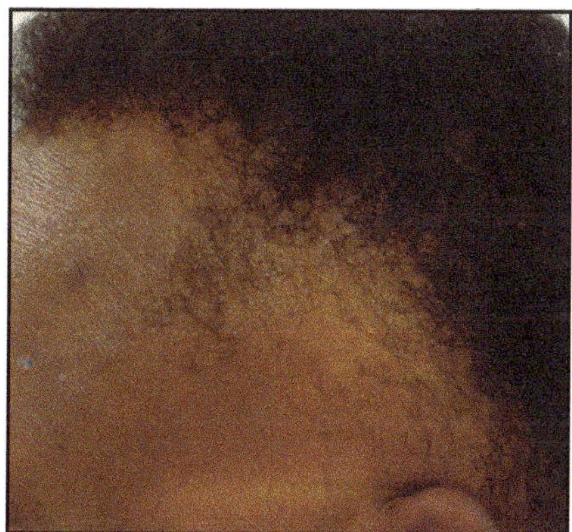

Figure 11B) Example of FFA – Sideburn Involvement

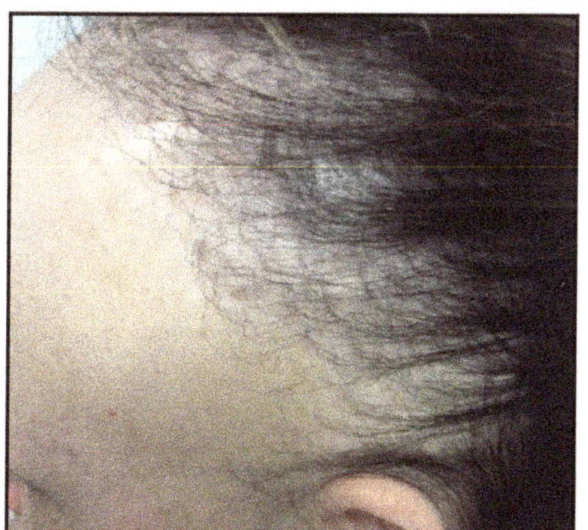

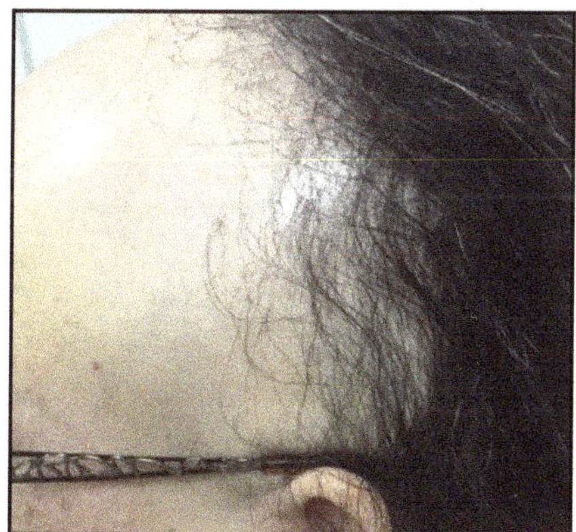

Figure 11B) Frontal Fibrosing Alopecia Progression from 2014 to 2016

Upon examination with a hand-held trichoscope, I discovered there was loss of hair follicle openings with redness and scaling around the follicles in several areas along Susan's frontal hairline (Fig. 11C). A small 4-mm punch biopsy was taken at the edge of the hair loss, where the redness and scaling around the follicles were present, indicating the FFA was active in that area. The biopsy returned with findings of lymphocytes (a type of inflammatory cell) with loss off sebaceous or oil glands and a decreased number of follicles with fibrosis (or scar tissue). The damage to the follicular structure differentiates between FFA and a non-scarring condition such as Traction Alopecia (TA). In TA, the "fringe sign" or a remnant of significantly short hairs along the margin of the hair loss, is usually present in front of the area of hair loss (Fig. 11D). The biopsy confirmed FFA rather than Pseudopelade, a similar scarring alopecia that lacks the element of active inflammation around the hair follicles.

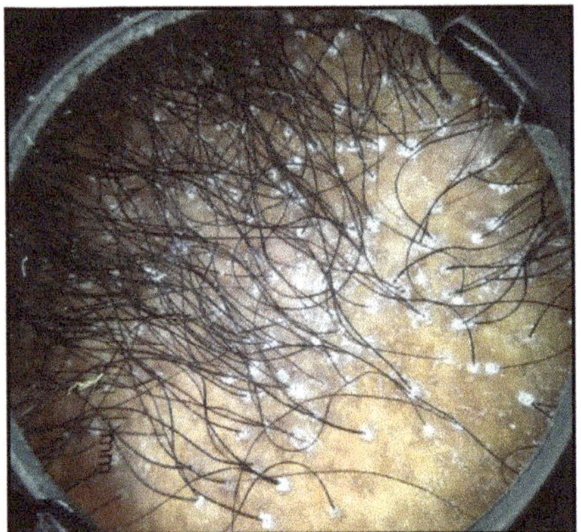

Figure 11C) Dermoscopy of FFA

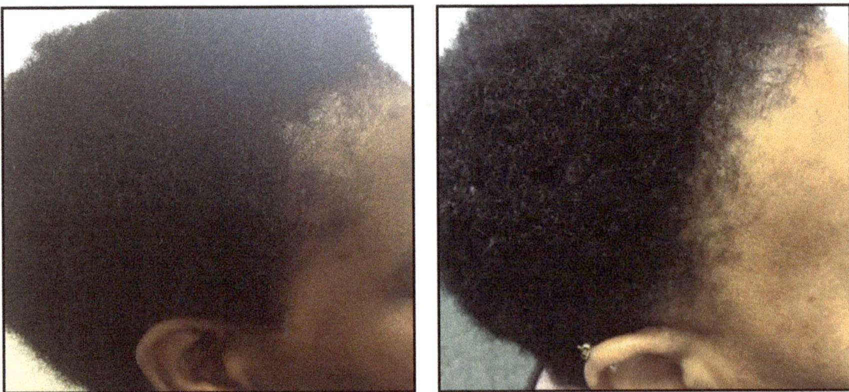

Figure 11D) Example of Traction Alopecia vs. Early Frontal Fibrosing Alopecia

TREATMENT OF FFA

In all scarring alopecias, treatment will not result in significant re-growth of the hair loss. The goal of treatment in all forms of LPP is to stop the progression of the disease and alleviate symptoms of discomfort. My first line of therapy for mild LPP is a combination of topical steroid formulation and steroid injections. Decreased redness and scaling around the follicles, symptoms, and slowed progression of hair loss should be seen by the three-month follow-up appointment. At that time, steroid use can then be tapered. The corticosteroid injections, along the area of active disease, can add effectiveness to the topical steroid treatment because it delivers the anti-inflammatory treatment to the deeper areas of the scalp.

If a patient has not responded within three months to combination steroid therapy, or the hair loss is progressing rapidly, my second line of treatment is hydroxychloroquine. This is an anti-malarial drug that has proven effectiveness in small clinical trials. It can rarely cause an eye condition called retinopathy. A complete eye exam by an optometrist should be done before starting therapy to create a baseline for monitoring the eyes every six to 12 months while on therapy. The benefit of hydroxychloroquine may be evaluated after at three months of therapy and a complete blood count is periodically done as it can rarely decrease the white blood cell count.

Oral antibiotics may also be prescribed in the treatment of FFA or LPP. Even though this is not a disease caused by an infection, antibiotics are helpful because of their anti-inflammatory effects. Minoxidil is also recommended to thicken residual small vellus hairs by lengthening the anagen or growing phase of the hair cycle.

Susan's story has become more common, so much so that researchers believe there is a worldwide epidemic of FFA the cause of which is not yet known. At the 2015 World Congress of Hair Research, several researchers presented theories around sunscreen or moisturizer use as possible contributory factors, given the location of hair loss.[38]

The rise in incidence of autoimmune scarring alopecias parallels the larger epidemic of many autoimmune diseases affecting millions in the U.S. and around the world today. A greater understanding of the autoimmune response is needed to prevent and treat hair loss as well as improve total body health and wellness.

---

38 Aldoori N, Dobson K, Holden CR, McDonagh AJ, Harries M, & Messenger AG. Frontal fi-brosing alopecia: possible association with leave-on facial skin care products and sun-screens; a questionnaire study. *J Dermatol.* 2016 Oct;175(4):762–767.

DISSECTING CELLULITIS OF THE SCALP
(DRAINING BOILS)

WHAT IS DISSECTING CELLULITIS OF THE SCALP?

Dissecting Cellulitis of the Scalp (DCS), also known as Hoffman's disease, is a rare primary scarring alopecia, and most commonly affects men of color in the second to fourth decade of life. Hoffman, a dermatologist, named and described the disease over a century ago in 1907. Its cause is unknown, but is related to the plugging of hair follicles called follicular occlusion, and resulting accumulation of inflammatory factors like TNF (Tumor Necrosis Factor). It has a similar pathophysiology as three other conditions: acne conglobata, hidradenitis suppuritiva, and pilonidal cysts—and the four together are sometimes called the "follicular occlusion tetrad." This is because in all four, the hair follicle or pore becomes clogged with keratin, a skin protein. Dilation follows causing inflammation, secondary bacterial infections, and resultant abscesses. Repeated episodes of inflammation and infection result in sinus tracts, scarring, and alopecia. FYI: Acne conglobate is a severe form of cystic acne covering the face, back, and chest. Hidradenitis suppurativa, is a similar inflammatory condition to DCS but occurs in the armpits and groin and pilonidal cysts of the groin.

A PATIENT'S EXPERIENCE WITH DCS

Rodney, a 31-year-old African American man, came to my office with active symptoms of DCS. He had been diagnosed with the condition four years earlier. At that time, he had a few small nodules that ranged in size from 5 mm to about 2 cm.

However, this visit marked his second relapse, and his pain and itching were more severe than previous episodes. His scalp was now covered with painful nodules from the crown to the nape of his scalp. The nodules were soft and boggy and drained pus with light pressure. Gentle pressure at one nodule caused drainage at another lesion, indicating that sinuses had formed deep into the scalp to create interconnecting abscesses. Small areas of scar tissue and permanent hair loss had occurred throughout the affected areas as well. Not only was Rodney in a significant amount of pain this time around, but he was very distressed about this appearance. He had draining sinus tracts between inflamed nodules and evidence of destruction of the hair follicles. He experienced itching and burning around the nodules in addition to extreme tenderness.

TREATMENT OF DCS

During Rodney's visit four years prior, a 4-mm punch biopsy that was taken from one of the active areas revealed a band of neutrophils (a type of inflammatory cell) in the deep dermis and subcutaneous tissue. The discharge from one nodule was cultured and identified as *Staphlococcus aureus*. At that time, he was treated with topical steroids and steroid injections, as well as a two-month course of Doxycycline for the staph infection. Rodney also used antiseptics daily to clean the infected area and avoided oil-based hair products. Our efforts resulted in remission of symptoms but obviously, no cure because now he was back again and so was his DCS — with a vengeance. I felt a new approach definitely had to be taken.

We began Rodney's treatment this time with oral and injected steroids immediately to reduce inflammation and to get the inflammation and progression under control. Because the disease had progressed to involve multiple areas of the scalp, Rodney agreed to a course of isotretinoin, an oral retinoid, which is frequently prescribed for severe nodulocystic acne but has been found to show significant improvement in DCS.[39] Isotretinoin suppresses the activity of the sebaceous or oil gland and is anti-inflammatory. It is a powerful medication and requires monitoring with blood tests to monitor liver function and cholesterol and triglycerides and monthly pregnancy tests in women. He agreed to return monthly during the one-year course of therapy. The Isotretinoin is usually continued for several months after the DSC appears to be in remission.

---

39 Koudoukpo C, Abdennader S, et al. Dissecting cellulitis of the scalp: a retrospective study of 7 cases confirming the efficacy of oral isotretinoin. *Ann Dermatol Venereol.* 2014 Aug-Sep;141(8-9):500–506.

For patients with more severe and resistant DCS, there are newer therapies that can offer hope for long-term remission and via blocking a key inflammatory factor driving TNF, like Humira or Remicade. These drugs suppress the immune system by blocking the activity of TNF, which can cause inflammation and contribute to the development of multiple conditions including psoriasis. We published a case success in the *Journal of Drugs in Dermatology*[40]

of a patient with resistant DCS that continued to flare despite multiple rounds of antibiotics, isotretinoin, and surgical excision. The patient was treated with an 80-mg loading dose and then 40 mg every other week. By the second month, some of the nodules resolved, pain diminished, and there was some hair re-growth. By the fifth month, all of the nodules resolved and there was significant hair re-growth. Very early treatment could well lead to prevention of chronic inflammation and scarring.

It has yet to be determined whether a prolonged use of TNF blockers as sole therapy results in actual resolution of sinus tracts. Another question is can therapy with TNF blockers be economically justified, as the treatments average upwards of $60,000 USD/year, and obtaining insurance coverage for them can be challenging, as the TNF blockers are not yet FDA approved for DCS.

In the case of a patient who does not respond well to medical treatments, the hair follicles can be reduced either surgically by scalp excision with skin grafting or with laser-assisted hair removal. With skin grafting, a split thickness skin graft is taken from another part of the body and is grafted to the scalp. A split thickness skin

---

40 Sukhatme SV, Lenzy YM, Gottlieb AB. Refractory dissecting cellulitis of the scalp treated with adalimumab. *J Drugs Dermatol.* 2008 Oct;7(10):981–983.

graft removes the entire epidermis, or outer layer of the skin, and a part of the dermis underneath. These grafts can create a clean skin surface for large areas. However, the hair loss is permanent, and the graft area is often lighter or darker than the surrounding skin, presenting a cosmetic challenge. The 1064-nm Nd:YAG laser, which is also used for facial laser hair removal in skin of color, may provide an alternate method of hair removal with less associated side effects. These methods of hair reduction have been successful at preventing further flares, but there is no chance of hair regrowth.

DCS is not life threatening, but can be debilitating because it is chronic and can result in relapsing despite treatment. The possibility of total cure is very poor. Complications can include squamous cell carcinoma, permanent hair loss, and marginal keratitis (an inflammation of the cornea that causes redness), sensitivity to light, and pus. Despite the poor prognosis, however, Rodney was very motivated to complete a treatment plan and to do all we could to stop his symptoms and arrest the progression of scarring and hair loss.

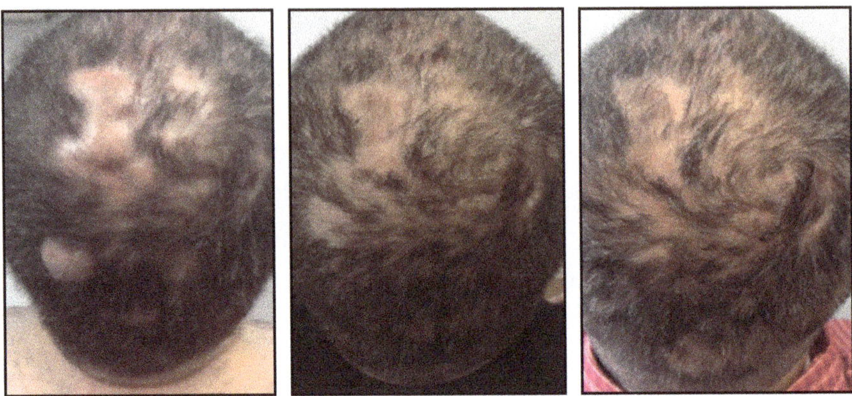

Figure 12) Left, DCS Pre-Treatment   Middle, Two Months on Humira   Right, Five Months on Humira

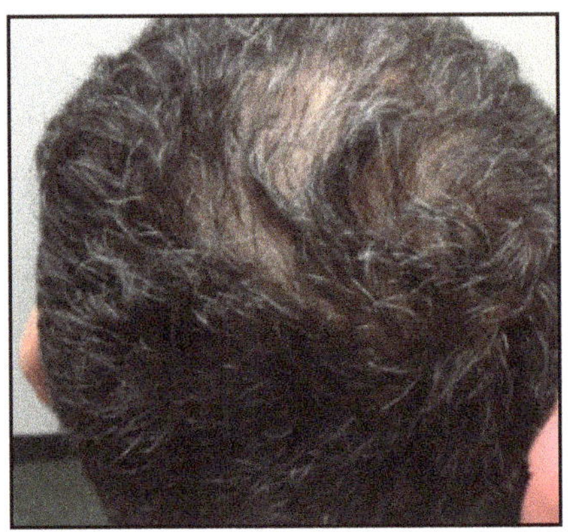

Figure 11C) Dermoscopy of FFA

FOLLICULITIS DECALVANS
(ITCHY & TENDER CRUSTED PATCHES)

WHAT IS FOLLICULITIS DECALVANS?

Folliculitis Decalvans (FD) is a long-term inflammatory condition of the scalp and is approximately 11 percent of all cases of scarring hair loss. Though very rare, FD occurs in young and middle-aged adults. It is seen more often in men than women and affects African American and Latino men more often than Caucasians. The exact cause of FD is unknown but it is associated with chronic inflammation from *Staphlococcus aureus*. It is believed that an immune deficiency is involved, as healthy skin also contains a small amount of *S. aureus* without the body reacting negatively to it. FD is not usually hereditary but there are rare reports of it affecting members of the same family. Some of its symptoms include itchy and painful scalp but in some cases, there may be no discomfort from the disease at all.

A PATIENT'S EXPERIENCE WITH FD

Ryan, a 22-year-old Hispanic male, came to my office because of burning and itching, a feeling of tightness in his scalp, and patchy hair loss. He described scaly scabs and crusts on his scalp that would sometimes bleed (Fig. 13). There was no family history of FD. He estimated that his symptoms had lasted more than one year, and the fear that he was "losing his hair" prompted him to seek medical treatment. He was wearing a tight cap to hide his thinning hair.

Examination of Ryan's scalp revealed multiple scaly plaques throughout his scalp that were tender, crusted, and a yellow-grey color. The redness and inflammation were more prominent at the crown and back of his head and there were small, irregular patches of hair loss at the crown of his scalp. The inflammation clearly involved the hair follicles and pressure on the swollen ones caused them to drain pus. Several of the hair follicles in the back were dilated and "tufted." Tufted means that the follicle has been damaged from chronic infection. Five to twenty hairs will emerge from a single follicle after it finally heals and forms one enlarged orifice. When this does happen, it gives the appearance of toothbrush bristles or doll hair with multiple hairs or bristles coming from one opening or pore. Eventually these hairs will fall out as the follicle is completely destroyed and becomes scarred. Ryan had no symptoms in any other hair bearing areas of the body, but he did have a history of staph infection following an injury to his leg in high school.

My suspicion of FD was confirmed by culturing a swab from the pus discharged from an inflamed follicle, and a nasal swab. Both were positive for *S. aureus*. A high neutrophil (a type of white blood cell) count was present as well, which is further confirmation of FD. I conducted a skin scraping for fungus, which can sometimes look similar to FD but it was negative. Last but not least, the results of a punch biopsy that is required to confirm the diagnosis revealed destruction of the sebaceous or oil glands with damage to the covering sheath of the follicle at the root. There were no sinus tracts between follicles, as is commonly seen in Dissecting Cellulitis (DCS).

TREATMENT OF FD

Because Ryan was uncomfortable with the itching and pain, my first treatment included topical and injected steroids to reduce inflammation and itching. Ryan used the topical cream twice a day with steroid injections into the affected area scheduled every six weeks. Once the inflammation was under control, our treatment goal included the elimination of *S. aureus*. Unlike ordinary Staph infections, short courses of antibiotics will not cure FD. Oral antibiotics, including doxycycline, and a combination of clindamycin plus rifampin can be effective in eliminating *S. aureus*. Doxycycline can be taken for a longer period of time without major side effects and long-term, low-dose use can prevent a relapse of symptoms. Hair restoration surgery is not a good option because of the chronic infection and ability for frequent flares seen in FD. It is only rarely considered, and only after several years with no symptoms of the disease.

Ryan had been very distressed about the inflammation and thinning of his hair. I assured him that although we do not expect hair regrowth, treatment could be expected to slow or stop the progression of the disease as well as further hair loss. We also discussed the fact that bacteria can grow in a warm, moist place, and wearing a bandana or hat for long periods of time can be a problem, as it could make it easier for bacteria to grow. Headgear must be kept clean and sterilized, and exposing the scalp to air will help facilitate the optimal environment for the scalp healing.

FD is a rare condition, so there are few studies to determine specific treatment and its course is unpredictable. FD may eventually stop on its own or "burn out," but patients often continue to have symptoms for many years. It is a condition which almost always requires continuous, long-term monitoring and treatment, and no permanent cure is known. Ryan was very motivated to participate in long-term treatment and was successful in relieving his symptoms and halting the hair loss after about four months. He continues to use topical steroids three times weekly in an effort to prevent recurrence of the inflammation.

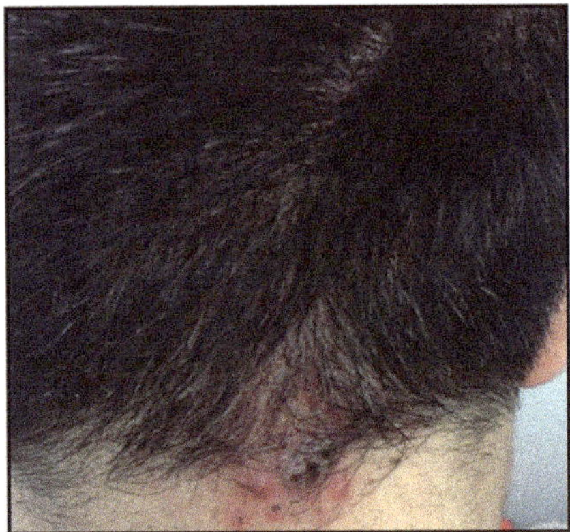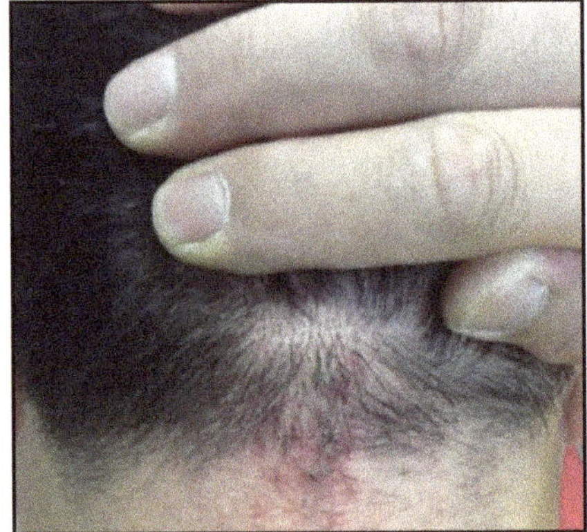

Figure 13) Folliculitis Decalvans at Diagnosis After 6 Months Combination Therapy

ACNE KELOIDOSIS NUCHAE & PSEUDOFOLLICULITIS BARBAE
(RAZOR BUMPS)

WHAT IS ACNE KELOIDOSIS NUCHAE?

Acne Keloidosis Nuchae (AKN) is a chronic scarring condition most common in African American men with a male-to-female ratio of at least 20:1. A 1997 study of 453 football players found that AKN is prevalent among male athletes of African descent, affecting more than 13 percent of players. The name Acne Keloidosis Nuchae was given to this condition in 1872. It begins with a mild inflammation and infection in and around the hair follicles, and its chronic and recurring nature leads to the formation of scars. The long-term infection can be painful, as well as distressing as scarring becomes visible. Contrary to its name, AKN is not true acne, and though the scarring causes elevated scars, a biopsy will show it is not actual keloid formation. True acne results from pores becoming clogged and forming "blackheads."

This is not common in AKN. The lesions tend to occur several days after shaving the area or getting a close haircut. It is thought that the coarse, curly hair re-enters the skin and becomes ingrown, causing irritation and inflammation. The ingrown hairs, however, do not fully account for the development of AKN. Irritation from shirt collars, chronic low-grade bacterial infection, autoimmunity, and some types of medication have also been suggested as contributing to the condition.

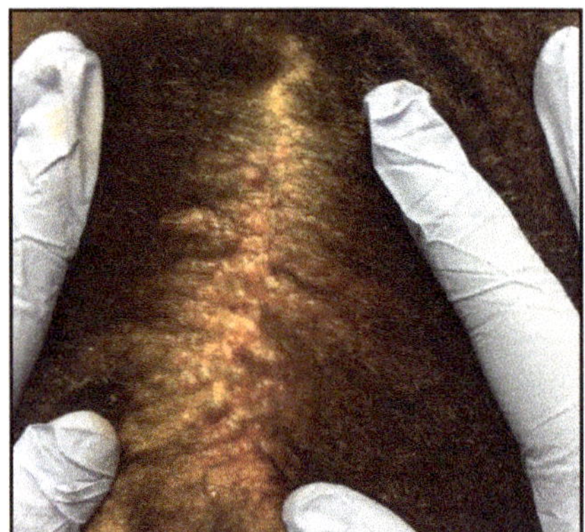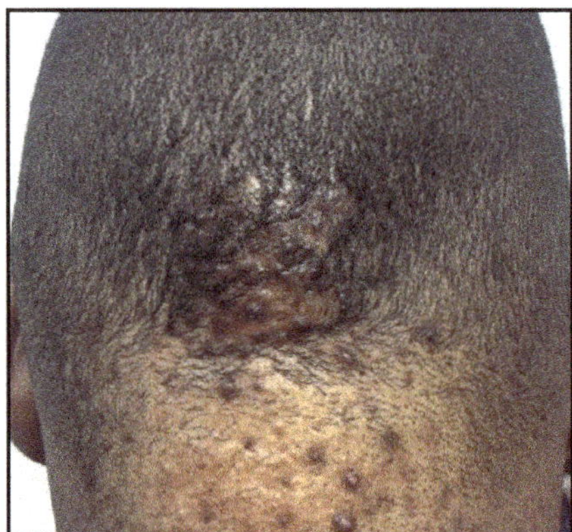

Figure 14A) and Figure 14B) Acne Keloidalis Nuchae in African American Men

A PATIENT'S EXPERIENCE WITH KN

Robert, a 40-year-old African American athlete, came to my office with inflamed bumps on the back of his scalp and neck. He complained that it was difficult to get the close-shaved haircut he was used to wearing because of hard, tender bumps at the hairline extending up the back of his scalp and down the back of his neck. Robert believed the lesions had been there for three years or more, and the itching and pain seemed worse to him immediately after a haircut. The back of Robert's scalp and neck was infected with more than 50 tiny dome-shaped, hard bumps called keloidal papules (Fig.

14A). A few tufted hairs were present where 20 or more hairs protruded from a single hair follicle, indicating an advanced stage of follicular damage. Intermingled with the tufts were small patches of scarring where the follicles were completely absent. There were also larger keloid-like scarred bumps at the nape of the scalp where chronic AKN had progressed. Robert asked if the infection could have been caused by non-sterilized clippers. I assured him that this is a myth and was not a factor in his condition.

TREATMENT OF ACNE KELOIDOSIS NUCHAE

I began treatment by addressing the inflammation and infection. A steroid cream in combination with the topical retinoid tretinoin was applied to the affected area twice daily, along with clindamycin, a topical antibiotic to heal the infection. Clobetasol is a super potent steroid that works by constricting blood vessels, inhibiting cell growth, and stimulating the production of enzymes that decrease inflammation. In addition to the topical treatments, I injected a steroid directly into the affected area to reduce the size and firmness of the papules. We also discussed practical ways Robert could alleviate the inflammation. Clothing or athletic gear that rubbed the area would be avoided. Also, I recommended discontinuing close haircuts that can facilitate ingrown hairs. Cleaning the affected area with a benzoyl peroxide wash and avoiding heavy oils would also aid in clearing the infection.

The problem of ingrown hairs can also occur in the beard, which creates a similar condition called Pseudofolliculitis barbae (PFB). Close shaving can result in the end of the hair reentering the skin and causing inflammation (Fig. 14C). The same treatment applies for this condition in the beard as Acne KN (AKN) of the scalp. There is no association between the two conditions. A patient may have either one or both.

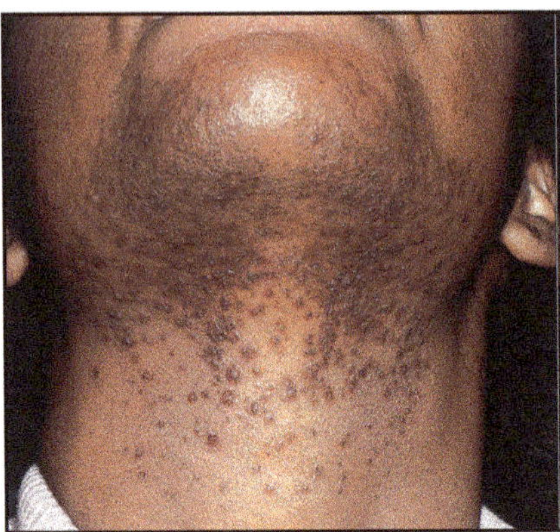

Figure 14C) Pseudofolliculitis Barbae

In severe cases of chronic AKN and PFB, more aggressive treatments may be used. Cryotherapy is the process of freezing the affected area for 20 seconds, allowing it to thaw, and then freezing again one minute later. Laser therapy monthly for four months can improve appearance and prevent the formation of additional lesions. Excision and surgical removal of scar tissue requires eight to 10 weeks of healing. The patient may have to wear a collar to prevent movement of the neck. Scarring and recurrence of lesions can occur after surgery, but generally the site is smaller and flatter than the original affected area.

After about four months of treatment with steroids, retinoids, and antibiotics, Robert's condition had improved. There was no sign of infection, and the redness and irritation had subsided. We discussed the fact that AKN is a chronic condition that is likely to recur. When the lesions first appear, it is important to begin treatment immediately to relieve discomfort and avoid any further scarring. Although Robert had been depressed about the appearance of disfiguring scars at the back of his scalp, he was relieved to experience successful healing with persistent treatment, cleansing, and avoiding mechanical irritation to the area.

DISCOID LUPUS ERYTHEMATOSUS
(SCALP & SKIN LUPUS)

WHAT IS DISCOID LUPUS ERYTHEMATOSUS?

Discoid Lupus Erythematosus (DLE) is an autoimmune condition of the skin with the development of inflammation and scarring that commonly affects the scalp, face, and sometimes other parts of the body. DLE is two to three times more common in women than men, and slightly more frequent in African Americans than in Caucasians and Asians. A small percentage of patients with DLE, about 16%, will develop Systemic Lupus Erythematosus, a more serious form of Lupus that affects the internal organs. The first symptoms of DLE usually appears before the age of 40, and continues intermittently throughout life, although about one-half of patients may achieve complete remission from symptoms over many years. Research suggests that smoking makes DLE worse. Even second-hand smoke can have a negative effect on the condition. In rare cases, chronic lesions of DLE can develop into skin cancer. Dark-skinned patients may be more prone to this because of the loss of pigmentation in the lesion, chronic inflammation, and sun damage. Squamous cell carcinoma is the most common form of skin cancer, which can develop into DLE and is more common in men with early age of onset, who use tobacco and have experienced lesions on the lips.

A PATIENT'S EXPERIENCE WITH DLE

Sandra, a 42-year-old African American woman, came to my office with a patchy, scaly rash throughout her scalp. Most of the spots were about 1 cm in size, slightly raised, and irregular in shape. Early evidence of scarring included minimal hair loss with depressed white patches in the center of a few of the plaques that had spread outward and become darker at the edges (Fig. 15A). Hair follicles in the affected areas were enlarged and plugged. There was also involvement in the bowl-shaped part of her outer ears called the "concha". Sandra said the rash had been present for about two years, and would itch and burn at times. She told me that she had just returned from a trip to Aruba and felt her symptoms had gotten worse while on vacation. The rash on Sandra's scalp was definitely characteristic of DLE. I asked her if any of her family members had symptoms similar to hers because, while it is rare for more than one family member to have lupus, it is believed that some families carry a gene that increases risk for developing the disease. Sandra couldn't recall anyone in her family that had any kind of symptoms similar to hers, however. Through several tests, I was able to classify Sandra's condition as "localized DLE," a milder form in which only the head and neck are affected.

DLE is classified as "widespread" when other areas, such as the cheeks, nose, and hands are affected, and these patients are more likely to develop SLE and experience more difficulty in treatment. These more difficult cases are sometimes associated with Raynaud's phenomenon or chilblains. Raynaud's phenomenon is a condition caused by constriction of small arteries, especially when exposed to cold or stress, producing numbness and tingling in the fingers and toes. In Raynaud's the affected areas turn red, white, and blue. Chilblains is pain caused by inflammation of the small blood vessels in response to sudden warming after exposure to the cold. Sandra also had concerns about her circulation and mentioned that she was always careful to wear gloves and boots in the winter. I ordered laboratory screening, including an anti-nuclear antibody (ANA) test, complete blood cell count, renal function, urinalysis, and rheumatoid factor. These negative results further confirmed that Sandra's lupus was limited to DLE without systemic involvement.

TREATMENT FOR DLE

My goals in treatment were to help Sandra improve her appearance by controlling the existing lesions, limit scarring, and to prevent development of further plaques. Sandra applied a topical steroid to the affected area to reduce inflammation. Topical steroids for the scalp are available in solutions, lotions, oils, or foams. The active lesions were injected with triamcinolone acetonide, a corticosteroid that penetrates deeper than the topical steroid application by the patient. I encouraged Sandra to follow her treatment regimen carefully as response varies from several weeks to several months. Some patients who are resistant to steroid therapy or who have more widespread involvement may require additional treatment. Hydroxychloroquine, an antimalarial medication taken orally, has been shown to decrease symptoms in multiple autoimmune conditions and prevent progression of DLE to SLE. The American Academy of Ophthalmology recommends an eye exam before taking antimalarial drugs. Removing scarred lesions is possible, but only done very rarely. This can result in reactivation of inactive lesions. Laser therapy is also used rarely for the same reason.

Sandra responded well to steroid therapy. After three months, she was symptom free with no signs of further progression of her scalp lesions. Her scalp showed signs of early hair regrowth. Scarring caused by lupus is different from other scarring alopecias where re-growth is usually not possible. In addition to her treatment, I informed Sandra that all varieties of lupus are considered photosensitive. Therefore, it was important that she avoid or limit sun exposure. I advised her to limit her sun exposure to early morning or late afternoon.

A wide-brimmed hat to protect the face and clothing containing sun protective factor (like those available at www.Coolibar.com) to protect the skin are necessary. If you can see through the shirt or blouse you're wearing, then sunlight can get through to your skin. Sunglasses and a sunscreen with a sun protection factor (spf) of 30 or higher should be re-applied every two–three hours. This will help to protect exposed skin.

Follow-up appointments are important. In Sandra's case, regular follow-up visits were made to check laboratory studies, to assess any changes, and to address any questions or symptoms that concerned her.

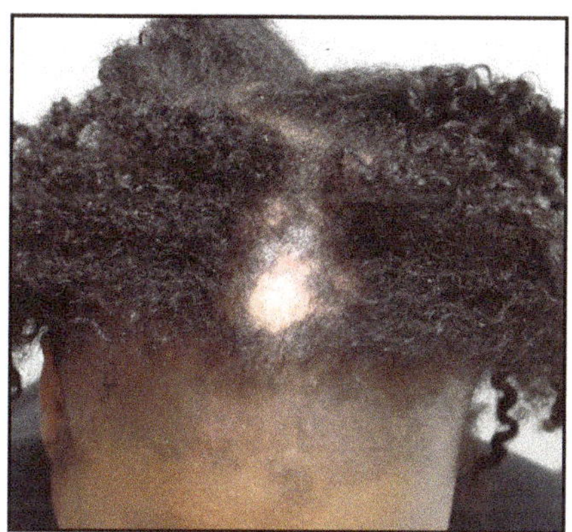

Figure 15A) Example of Discoid Lupus Erythematosus

SEBORRHEIC DERMATITIS
(DANDRUFF)

WHAT IS SEBORRHEIC DERMATITIS?

Seborrheic Dermatitis (SD) is a common condition that commonly affects the scalp and skin, where symptoms may range from dry flakes (aka, dandruff) to yellow, greasy scales with background skin redness on the skin. It occurs more frequently in newborns and adults ages 30 to 60, and is slightly more commonly in men than women. In addition to the scalp, SD often appears on the face and chest, regions of the skin with the most active sebaceous, or oil, glands. In addition to oily skin, SD is also associated with an inflammatory response to the natural yeast on the skin called Malassezia. SD can be more severe with changes in temperature and remission commonly occurs in the summer. Stress has been attributed with flares of SD as well as a number of inflammatory skin and scalp conditions.

Dandruff, the mildest form of SD, affects 15 percent to 20 percent of the population, which makes it the second most common inflammatory skin condition, next to acne. It occurs in people of all races, but is frequently seen in African Americans possibly due to variations in shampooing frequency. Noticeable light patches on the skin, called Hypopigmentation, is a manifestation of SD in African Americans. SD is not completely preventable or curable, but it is highly controllable with the proper treatment and hair and skin care.

SD may be associated with other conditions, including Parkinson's disease, depression, HIV/AIDS, alcoholic pancreatitis, congestive heart failure, eating disorders, epilepsy, and diabetes. It can also occur simultaneously with other forms of alopecia, especially Central Centrifugal Cicatricial Alopecia (CCCA, see Chapter 8).

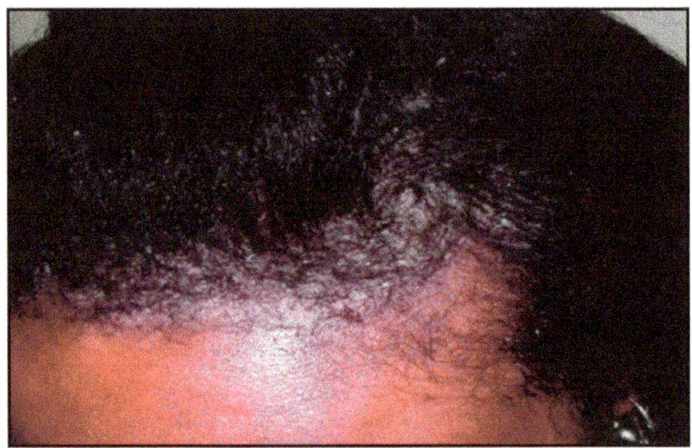

Figure 16 – Seborrheic Dermatitis

A PATIENT'S EXPERIENCE WITH SD

Hailey, a 38-year-old African American woman, came to my office because of dry, itchy scalp and dryness and flaking in between her eyebrows and along the sides of her nose. Hailey had experienced similar episodes since her early 30's, and found that her symptoms were worse in the winter and early spring when the weather turned dry and cold. She had been controlling her symptoms with over-the-counter (OTC) medicated dandruff shampoos, including Head & Shoulders, Selsun Blue, and Neutrogena T-Gel, but this year her "dry scalp" was particularly resistant to these treatments. Upon examination, it became apparent that Hailey was suffering from SD. Her scalp had thick, adherent patches of white/yellow "build-up" or scales throughout her scalp (Fig. 16). The affected areas on her face were red with dry, white scales, and there was evidence that her scalp was extremely itchy, as she had scratched her temples to a point that the skin was now slightly thickened, a feature that we call lichenification, since it likens the rough texture and thickness that is present on the bark of a tree. Hailey was very embarrassed and anxious about her condition and had stopped wearing black clothing because the contrast made the scales which fell on her clothes more visible. I assured her it was not due to poor hygiene, and by carefully following the treatment plan, we would get the condition under control.

TREATMENT FOR SD

Hailey began her treatment with Ketoconazole 2%, a prescription antifungal dandruff shampoo that she could use one to two times weekly (I vary the prescribed frequency of use based on the severity of the scaling and itching) on the scalp and daily as a face wash. Most people make the mistake of only leaving a medicated shampoo on the scalp for a short period of time as they would a non-medicated shampoo, not allowing it time to work. It is important to take time for the medicated shampoo to sit and allow the treatment to have full effect. Here are the steps that I recommend to achieve maximum benefit from your therapeutic shampoo:

- Apply medicated shampoo to dry scalp and allow it to sit for 10 minutes.

- Wet hair and lather scalp area only (meaning do not pull the lather all the way through the hair shaft and ends, gently massaging to loosen scales.

- Rinse, and follow with a moisturizing, hydrating shampoo to concentrate the hair shaft and ends.

- Rinse, and apply a topical steroid if needed to control itching (examples are Clobetasol, Fluocinonide or Fluocinolone). They are available as ointment, oils, solution, or cream formulations. Then style as usual.

- Finally, apply a deep conditioner and sit under a steamer for 15-20 minutes or apply a warm towel and then a shower cap to create a "steam effect."

- Repeat the above regimen as needed until desired control is achieved.

In babies, SD is commonly called "cradle cap." It appears in babies three months or younger, and usually resolves completely before they are one year old. A dandruff shampoo is generally not recommended for infants, as it could irritate their delicate skin. The affected area can be massaged with a gentle oil (like extra virgin olive oil) and brushed with a baby hairbrush to release the scales. Shampoo the scalp daily with baby shampoo and warm water. Babies can also develop SD in the diaper area, which is commonly accompanied by yeast overgrowth called Candida and is treated with an anti-fungal cream.

Once Hailey resolved this flare, she returned to using over-the-counter anti-dandruff shampoos, which contain zinc pyrithione or selenium sulfide as key ingredients for maintenance. It is not uncommon for the ingredients in a medicated shampoo to be effective for a time and then lose their effectiveness over time. Therefore, I often recommend alternating between two different types of OTC medicated shampoos. These milder shampoos can also be used as a face wash and then rinsed off completely and followed by a moisturizer. I advised her to avoid products that contain alcohol, like hair sprays and gels, as these can dry out the skin and sometimes exacerbate a SD flare. If eyelids show signs of scaling, they can be washed gently with a gentle cleanser and rinsed thoroughly. A warm compress may aid in removing scales. I also reminded her to resist scratching the affected areas as this can increase susceptibility to infection. When the scales are particularly thick and adherent to the scalp, I recommend an overnight treatment in which the patient massages jojoba or olive oil into the scalp, cover with a shower cap, then follow the above routine the following morning. Hailey schedules an appointment each year at the beginning of winter, which is when her flares are worst. She has managed her SD with good scalp and skin care for several years.

SCALP PSORIASIS
(THICK SCALY PLAQUES)

WHAT IS SCALP PSORIASIS?

Scalp psoriasis is a common skin disorder that presents with pink/salmon-colored plaques with an overlying thick, silvery scale. Psoriasis is often confused with Seborrheic Dermatitis (SD), but the causes and the appearance differ. In psoriasis, the scales are thicker and appear in well-defined patches, while in SD the scales are more diffuse and superficial. Often, patients with scalp psoriasis will also have thick, scaly plaques on the elbows, knees, hands, or feet. There may also be tiny pits or yellow patches on the fingernails. In many patients, both conditions tend to worsen when the weather turns cold and dry. A sub-type called Guttate Psoriasis with smaller, round, or "guttate" plaques can typically be seen in children following a Strep infection. Psoriasis currently affects 2 percent to 3 percent of the population, world-wide and about 7.5 million Americans. In psoriasis, the top layer of skin called the Stratum Corneum, matures in four days versus the normal rate of

28 days (7 times faster than normal), leading to the thickened or hyperkeratotic plaques. Contrary to common fears, psoriasis is not related to poor hygiene, and is not contagious. Between 50 percent and 80 percent of patients present with scalp involvement alone or in conjunction with involvement on other parts of the body.

A PATIENT'S EXPERIENCE WITH SCALP PSORIASIS

Janie, a 31-year-old Asian American female, came to my office concerned about her dry, flaky scalp. She was anxious and embarrassed to talk about her symptoms, which had been getting worse for over a year. Janie had thick, pink plaques throughout her scalp covered with silver-white flakes, similar to dandruff. Her scalp was very inflamed and somewhat tender as I carefully examined her. I noticed a few thick, pink, and scaly plaques on Janie's elbows and knees as well. There were also a few crusted sores from scratching where there had been intense itching. Janie said she could not sleep at times because the itching was so severe. In addition, there were a few small patches of hair loss. Right away I could tell that Janie was suffering from scalp psoriasis.

I began by reassuring Janie that scalp psoriasis is a common condition. While the exact cause of psoriasis remains elusive, it is largely due to a complex interaction between genetics and over-activity of a pro-inflammatory immune response. This response results in the skin cells turning over too quickly and the buildup of thick, scaly patches. Psoriasis is most common among Caucasians and less common in Asian and African populations. She was concerned about the small, irregular patches of hair loss, and I assured her that they should grow back with persistent treatment. Hair loss is a common complaint in individuals and with patients with scalp involvement, but Telogen Effluvium (see Chapter 2) due to the inflammatory process and trauma, caused by scratching of itchy lesions, are believed to be the cause in most of these cases.3 Few reports of scarring alopecia due to psoriasis have been published. There is no cure for psoriasis, but with consistent care it can be controlled, and the symptoms relieved.

TREATMENT FOR SCALP PSORIASIS

The most important consideration in treating scalp psoriasis topically is getting the medication to penetrate the thick scales on the scalp. The tar, selenium, and salicylic acid shampoos are designed to loosen the scales and reduce the itching. I prefer to use shampoos containing Ketoconazole or Ciclopirox in my regimens as a scalp-focused (versus hair shaft) treatment (see below). The hair shaft itself needs a gentle moisturizing shampoo, so caring for the scalp and caring for the hair will involve two different treatments.

Scalp medications are available in an oil, creams, ointments, or solutions, depending on your preference. I prescribed Fluocinolone oil for Janie, which is also available as DermaSmoothe® Scalp Oil. It is a corticosteroid that reduces inflammation and helps to loosen the plaques. The following steps can be followed two to three times weekly, depending on the severity. I like to limit the duration of corticosteroid use to no more than three weeks straight before taking a break to help prevent side effects.

Step 1: Fluocinolone oil is applied to the dry scalp and gently massaged to loosen scales. Do not use fingernails! Gentle rubbing will loosen plaques and prevent further irritation. Cover the scalp with a shower cap and leave the oil on overnight.

Step 2: The next day, apply medicated shampoo containing Ketoconazole or Ciclopirox to dry scalp for 10 minutes. Then wet your hair and lather the scalp only. This portion of the treatment concentrates on the scalp condition. Rinse after 10 minutes; then follow with a moisturizing, hydrating shampoo for the hair strands. I recommend **Shea Moisture African Black Soap Shampoo and Conditioner or Shampoo** when conducting clinical testing.

Step 3: Apply a leave-on topical steroid (like Clobetasol or Fluocinonide) to control itching. You can request the vehicle of your choice – ointment, solution, oil, cream, or spray.

Step 4: Follow with a deep conditioner.

Improvement with topicals can take six weeks or more. It is important to be consistent with your prescribed treatments and not get discouraged if you don't see immediate results. In very severe cases of scalp psoriasis, a corticosteroid can be injected (yes, with a tiny needle!) directly into the inflamed plaques on the scalp about every six weeks. UV light in the form of the excimer laser targeted directly to the affected area can also aid in improvement.

If there is insufficient improvement with the topical or light-based therapies or there is significant area of the body surface area (BSA) involved (typically >10%), systemic treatments either taken orally or via injections are typically the next line of attack. Methotrexate is often the first oral medication prescribed, which is taken once weekly and can help to decrease the thickness of the psoriasis plaques as well as the itching. Laboratory tests, including liver and kidney function, blood counts, and a pregnancy test, are checked prior to starting to Methotrexate, and these have to be monitored while on treatment. Methotrexate should be avoided in individuals with a history of liver disease. Therefore, a liver biopsy is generally recommended when a cumulative dose of 1.5 g of Methotrexate is reached. My personal practice is to avoid treating patients with Methotrexate for longer than one year to avoid this need. Once my patients have been on Methotrexate for one year with good control of the psoriasis, I often switch them to another category of systemic treatment for psoriasis called biologics.

The FDA has also approved a class of drugs called biologics for the treatment of psoriasis. Biologics are also called "biological response modifiers," because they interfere with the body's pro-immune response that prevents the rapid stratum corneum turnover that causes psoriasis. There are now many biologics on the market that target steps in the inflammatory cascade, reducing inflammation and altering the immune response Adalimumab (Humira®) or Etanercept (Enbrel®) inhibit tumor necrosis factor-alpha. Ustekinumab (Stelara®) interferes with Interleukin (IL)-12 and IL-23, Secukinumab (Cosentyx®) and Ixekinumab (Taltz®) block IL-17 and the newest biologic to market Guselkinumab (Tremfya®) inhibits IL-23-induced responses, including release of pro-inflammatory cytokines. Biologics are also used to treat other autoimmune disorders like rheumatoid arthritis and some cancers.

Janie responded well to the topical treatments I recommended. When I saw her eight weeks later, her symptoms had almost completely cleared. With the relief from intense itching, she was sleeping through the night. The small patches of alopecia showed signs of hair regrowth, and the moisturizing shampoo had restored the shine and softness to her hair. Janie scheduled a follow-up appointment for the beginning of winter when flares tend to be worse. Janie now felt equipped that she had a plan, the knowledge, and tools to manage her psoriasis successfully.

GOING NATURAL — TWO METHODS, ONE GOAL

There are two major methods for going natural, or discontinuing chemical relaxers: 1) transitioning out of the relaxer by cutting the hair over time or 2) performing a "big chop." When people aren't ready to radically change their longer to very short hair, they may choose to transition with heat-based styling. Alternatively, some people choose to "big chop," or cut off all relaxed hair at once.

METHOD ONE: THE SLOW TRANSITION

The benefit of transitioning over time is that women get to retain their length throughout the transition. During a transition, the previously relaxed hair is progressively cut off as your natural hair grows out.

Styling Transitioning Hair

In styling transitioning hair, the goal is to blend the new growth hair with the previously relaxed hair. One method of blending is via heat. Blow-drying, flat-ironing, and, more rarely, using pressing combs and curling irons, are just a few thermal heat methods that will help unrelaxed hair achieve a straightened look.

An alternative method of blending relaxed and natural hair is with curly set styles. Roller, flexi-rod, or perm rod sets are also methods of styling combination (natural and relaxed) hair. With less direct heat, these methods are useful for someone who is concerned about potential "heat damage," which can commonly occur with consistent use of thermal heat methods used to straighten natural hair. Between the two methods, direct heat and set styles, the latter is less damaging.

Still another option is the so-called "protective" style. Protective styles is the term used to describe styles that require minimal daily manipulation like braids, sew-in weaves, buns, etc. to give your own hair a "rest." I emphasize "so-called" because these styles are not always protective. Some of these styles could actually lead to *more* hair loss in several forms. Tight or even heavy braids or cornrows place excessive strain leading to inflammation on the hair follicle. Extension methods that utilize glues or adhesives can damage the scalp in the removal process or even cause contact dermatitis.[41] Hence, the word "protective" is often a misnomer. But as with anything, the benefit or risk depends on factors that a knowledgeable stylist could help you mitigate—frequency, tightness, length of time the styles stay in, etc.

---

41 Torchia D, Giorgini S, et al. Allergic contact dermatitis from 2-ethylhexyl acrylate contained in a wig-fixing adhesive tape and its 'incidental' therapeutic effect on alopecia areata. *Contact Dermatitis.* 2008 Mar;58(3):170–171.

Challenges of the Long Transition

One downside of the long transition is that it can be difficult to care for hair that is two different textures, as each texture requires different products, styling methods, and maintenance to help it be great. New growth hair tends to be very dry, while previously relaxed hair retains moisture because of the straightened shaft, so moisture balance tends to be difficult to maintain. Furthermore, the line of demarcation, the point where new growth and previously relaxed hair meet, is the most sensitive to breakage because it is the weakest portion of the hair shaft. Therefore, hair in transition can be challenging for someone to take care of on their own. Although a very skilled stylist can be helpful in the transition, it is still common to experience some breakage while the hair is transitioning.

Another challenge of transitioning from straight to natural hair is exercising. When you're using heat to style your hair, sweating from exercise can cause the new growth to revert back to the natural texture at the roots which, for some people, defeats the purpose of the straight look they are trying to achieve. Concern over "sweating out one's hair" has been identified in multiple studies as a barrier to achieving the 150 minutes of moderate intensity physical activity recommended by the Center for Disease Control and Prevention to maintain health.[42] Therefore, heat-based styling of natural hair has a higher risk of influencing someone to choose their "hair over health" due to not wanting to sweat out the style.

Heather Worthy and Desiree Williams explore this phenomenon in their recent book, "Love Affair With My Hair: Why Black Women

---

42 https://www.cdc.gov/physicalactivity/data/facts.htm

Cheat on Health."[43] Williams attained her doctorate in Physical Therapy and is a professor and former Miss Virginia. In "*Love Affair*," Williams and Worthy develop a 12-week fitness program that works around regular hair appointments. For example, the first few days after the hair appointment are filled with low-intensity workout plans that achieve results without causing excessive sweating. Then you increase your intensity as you get closer to the day of your next hair appointment. Williams and Worthy also incorporate rotational hair styles in their twelve-week plan. I recommend this book for any woman who is considering transitioning, but is also concerned about her exercise regimen. I'm happy that there is more literature on the market that addresses this very challenging issue women face when deciding what to do about their hair as they consider their own fitness. My own fitness goals were the reason I chose to utilize the second method, the "big chop", for going natural back in 2015.

METHOD TWO: THE BIG CHOP

"The Big Chop" is a method of cutting off all of the relaxed and heat-damaged hair in one single swoop. One benefit of this method is that one does not have to worry about caring for or styling two different hair textures. Another benefit is that the resultant style, affectionately referred to in the natural hair community as a TWA or "teeny weenie afro," can be easily worn as a "wash and go" and is a very exercise-friendly hairstyle. After a big chop, you don't have to worry about heat and straightening, which are great benefits. However, one potential challenge of cutting a significant amount of hair at one time is a more drastic change in your

---

43 http://www.amazon.com/Love-Affair-With-My-Hair/dp/1505575915

look of going from longer hair to shorter hair in a short period of time.

Depending on your geographical location, you may also experience pressure from outside sources, as employers have questioned the professionalism of natural hairstyles. This is definitely changing as natural hairstyles are gaining exposure nationally because of actresses like Viola Davis and Lupita Nyongo, and musicians like Layla Hathaway and India Arie. However, there are still some areas with more limited standards of professionalism. In places like this, employers may see straightened hair as somehow more professional than textured, natural hair. As a private business owner, I escaped this challenge in my journey.

MY STORY

When I relocated from Boston to where I currently live, I decided to transition out of relaxers (which I faithfully had professionally done every eight weeks or so since I was in the fifth grade) after I had my first experience of scalp burning and subsequent scabbing during and after my last relaxer application in August 2012. When I got home from that salon appointment and felt those scabs once I ran my fingers through my scalp, I was terrified, as I knew the scientific evidence around the increased risk of scarring alopecia with burning from relaxers. It was at that instance that I decided, NO MORE! I had actually been thinking about "going natural" for some time, mainly to see what the process would be like since I commonly recommended it to patients who were dealing with certain types of hair loss or excessive breakage. I began to transition in that fall and I found a new stylist who was comfortable managing natural hair. I still remember it like it was yesterday when she cut my hair into an angled bob. I posted the pic on Facebook (the ultimate litmus test, right?) and the engagement of likes, hearts, and comments went through the roof. I was like, "OK, I can do this!"

For the next three years, I faithfully got my hair shampooed, blow-dried, and flat-ironed and kept it cut in a shoulder-length bob. It was gorgeous, full, and very healthy...or so I thought. My hair was shoulder length before the transition and since it remained straight due to thermally straightening it, no one really knew that my hair was natural unless I mentioned it. The first two summers of my transition posed challenges. If I went outside and did a major run or some other vigorous exercise, my blow out definitely got "sweated out." It was difficult to maintain a straight style that blended both textures. Although it wasn't a major issue, it was part of the reason that I decided to cut my hair enough to wear it in its natural texture, especially as I was getting more active with exercise.

One misconception people naturally have about transitioning is that they can retain their natural curl pattern despite using heat consistently. Although I had grown my hair for three years without a relaxer, I now needed to "big chop" the heat-damaged ends. Those ends would no longer curl when my hair was wet, in order to be able to wear my hair in a curly style or a "wash and go" without setting it on rollers or rods.

[As you're straightening your hair thermally, it's really hard to know where the relaxed hair ends and the natural hair begins. Your own natural hair may lose its curl because of heat damage. Since my heat-processed hair didn't curl up the way that my own hair does now, it's hard to know how long it would have taken me to grow out a fuller afro with the slow transition. I measured my progress mainly by how much I'd been cutting my hair, since it was growing while I was cutting it. Although I'd cut most of my relaxed hair away already, this didn't mean, however, that my hair was ready for a natural style such as the wash and go.]

Before the summer of 2015, I'd been inconsistent in my exercise. I might have exercised for 30 minutes two or three days a week, either on the elliptical machine or running. I wasn't completely sedentary, but I wasn't doing the optimal CDC recommendation of 150 minutes per week.[44] At the beginning of the summer of 2015, I decided that I wanted to really take my fitness to another level. I have a strong family history of obesity, which can sometimes be hereditary. Obesity is just one risk factor for many diseases like Diabetes, Hypertension, and High Cholesterol, which can lead to life-threatening consequences. Although can't do anything about our genetic makeup, I am aware that my actions can help increase or decrease certain genetic risks. So that summer, with my running and increased vigorous physical activity, my hair was not lasting as long as it had been during the winter, or prior summers when I hadn't been working out as hard.

At the beginning of June 2015, I decided that I was not going to use any more heat to style my hair. Throughout the summer I just had my hair done in roller set styles or perm rod sets. I had one thermal straightening that summer—I was speaking at the American Academy of Dermatology's summer meeting in August so I got my hair straightened. It wasn't that I thought that a curly hairstyle would not have been acceptable for that conference; I'd

---

44 The Center for Disease Control and Prevention recommends adults engage in
    150 minutes of vig-orous exercise a week to maintain their current weight or 250
    minutes per week to lose weight.

just learned from experience that roller sets on combination hair could be unpredictable. In the morning, sometimes I would have areas on the sides of my hair that I slept rough on inciting a little morning hairstyling stress. Therefore, for that meeting, since I was already a bit nervous about the talk, I didn't want to wake up and find that my hair was a mess. Straightening my hair for that conference eased my nerves a bit.

After the conference, I began planning for vacation and decided to get braids. I spoke earlier about braids as a so-called "protective style." I usually only get my hair braided for vacation, and then I keep the braids in only for a couple of weeks to decrease the amount of damage the added weight might do to my follicles. When I took those braids out, I decided to cut it.

Prior to the big chop, I went on Instagram and Pinterest and started to follow different pages focused on TWAs or ones featuring hairstyles I liked. (The easiest way to do this is to search for the hashtags #TWA, #BigChop, and #Natural Hair in the search tab.) I like to show my stylist the kind of style I am thinking about to ensure that we are on the same page.

I sent my stylist a couple of photos of styles that I was thinking of. The part that was unknown was what type of natural curl pattern I actually had. Although you have a photo of someone's hair that you like, there is no guarantee that it will look the same because you might not have the same curl pattern that they have. Some naturals use a curl typing system to describe the type of curl pattern they have (Fig. 18). If the person in the photo has a looser curl pattern and you have a tighter texture, it's not going to look the same because you have different textures.

Hair types

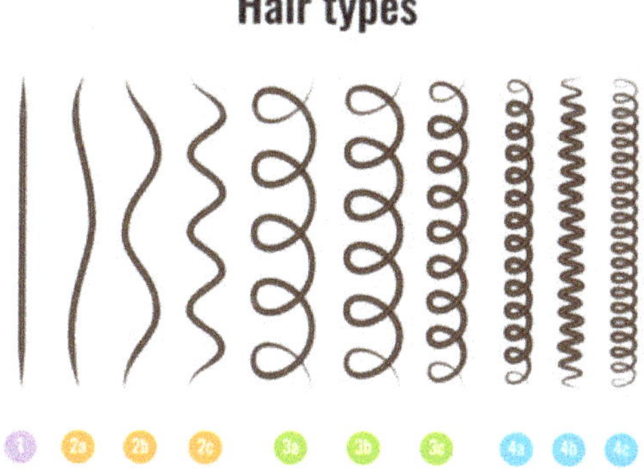

Figure 18-Curl Typing System
Credit: ID 118496038 © Aleksandra Nekrasova | Dreamstime.com

But what I didn't realize is that most of us have various different curl patterns in different parts of our hair. The back of my hair and edges have a much looser curl pattern than my crown, which is very coarse and very coily. And my sideburns are very fine. In choosing styles that fit me, I had to think about my different textures.

My next step was figuring out how I was going to wear it. Was I just going to wear it in an afro? Did I want to have some type of additional setting styling done to it? I decided to see one of my colleagues, Shea Moisture[45] beauty ambassador, Diane C. Bailey in Brooklyn, NY, to learn more about various styling options for my TWA. We tried several different methods, including the wash-and-go method, the curling sponge, and my favorite, the comb coiling technique. Comb coiling, she said, would give me a little bit

---

45 Shea Moisture is a Black-owned company that sells personal care and beauty products. Their products are organic and natural, and are sulfate and paraben-free. You can find out more at www.sheamoisture.com.

more curl definition — especially in the crown of my head, which as I mentioned, had a more coily texture. That section was coarse and did not have an apparent defined curl pattern like the edges and the back of my hair did. I soon found a local stylist, Shelia Vann who could maintain the comb coiling style for me. That is how I wore my hair for the first six to eight months after my big chop.

TWA's Professional Debut

I have found one of the great benefits of owning my own business is not having to worry about anyone else's ideas about what constitutes a professional hair style. Al-though I wanted to make sure that I looked professional before my patients or my customers, it certainly felt freeing to not have to worry about someone coming and telling me, "Oh, I don't think your hair looks professional." I doubted very seriously that a patient would tell me that, so that alleviated a bit of the stress I know some women feel when they are considering a transition to natural hair.

My first professional appearance after the big chop was actually a hugely important lecture that I was invited to give. I was selected to be a visiting professor at the Mayo Clinic in October 2015 to give a lecture on Ethnic Hair and Health Disparities in Dermatology. This was also my first professional debut of my new style. In the middle of my lesson about ethnic hair, I reached the section where I teach the information that I am discussing with you right now on natural hair and the TWA. I paused and said, "The style that I'm wearing today in the natural hair community is called a TWA, which stands for "teeny weeny afro." At the end of the talk, the chairman of the department stood up to ask a question and said, "I think your TWA looks fantastic." Everybody clapped in agreement. I responded, "Oh, you got the terminology!" It was really awesome. A style that I was still getting used to had given us a great teaching moment. And it was just affirming to me, as this was an environment which was not very diverse. They had one African American resident, but the rest of the department was non-Black. This was my first time trying out this style in an environment with people who had probably seen styles like mine, but had never been formally educated about what it took to achieve the style. These were dermatologists who needed to learn about the diversity of hair care practices, and my TWA broke the ice in a cross-cultural conversation.

TWA's Family Debut

Although I was nervous about debuting my hair to that audience, I was even more nervous about wearing my TWA around my own family, church and biological, for the first time. In our community, many older women do not seem to care for short, natural hair. When I first saw my own family, my aunt said, "Why you cut off all that pretty hair?" My family members were not used to the idea of someone wearing short, natural hair by choice. Of course, they had seen people's hair break off, resulting in the necessity of a shorter style. But they hadn't seen someone with a full, healthy head of hair choose to cut it off. That was pretty much unheard of. Once I explained my reasoning, she said, "Oh yeah, that makes sense." I had similar apprehensions about wearing my new style to church, but the reactions all around were positive.

I want to acknowledge that my hair journey may be unique in that the primary caretaker of my hair has been a professional stylist. Even when my hair was relaxed and transitioning, I'd always gone to a professional stylist regularly. My time with the stylist is my "me-time," and I still don't do my primary hair care myself. I don't generally wash my hair myself or take it from start to finish because I just enjoy being able to go and read a magazine or a book while having it styled. I know that this is a luxury. Many women manage their haircare themselves. Some are either unable to see a stylist regularly, or live in an area without ready access to a natural hair stylist.

Even with the additional challenges that some of my patients may face with their own natural hair transition, I would still encourage them, if possible, to go natural given the conflicting research finding of an association of relaxers with certain forms of hair loss. My mantra regarding the safety of hair styling practices is, "When in doubt, leave it out." In my opinion and experience, the benefits far outweigh the costs.

With natural hair, I'm able to work out as intensely as I please without worrying about "sweating out my style" and worrying if I will be able to get my hair together in a short period of time before I go to work. If I sweat, it's not a problem. I can just use a moisture mist to spritz it and I'm able to just go. That's been the most freeing thing about the whole process. Second, my natural hair has been really inspirational for my patients who are dealing with alopecia. For some time now, I have been encouraging my patients with various forms of hair loss to go natural. Many of them have shared with me that seeing me wear my hair in this aesthetic has helped them to make the choice regarding their own transition or chop.

This journey has also helped me get in touch with my natural texture. I didn't know what it was like because as far as I can remember, I have had my hair straightened, either chemically or thermally. Like many black women, I began to have my hair straightened in elementary school. Therefore, my natural hair journey has helped me to appreciate my hair for how it grows out of my head and enjoy it for what it is. Finally, through the choices I am making for my hair care like avoiding chemicals as well as frequent braiding or weaving and rotating various natural hairstyles (Fig. 19), I feel like I'm doing everything that I can possibly do to try to prevent the development of CCCA or Central Centrifugal Cicatricial Alopecia (see Chapter 10). There is a very strong family history of CCCA in my family with my mother, sister, several paternal aunts, cousins, and my grandmother all having that condition. Although having natural hair does not guarantee that I won't ever develop it, I at least feel like I'm doing my part.

Figure 19) My Rotation of Natural Hairstyles

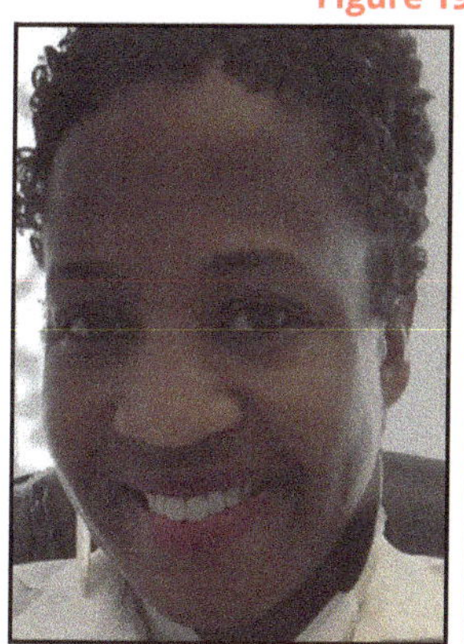 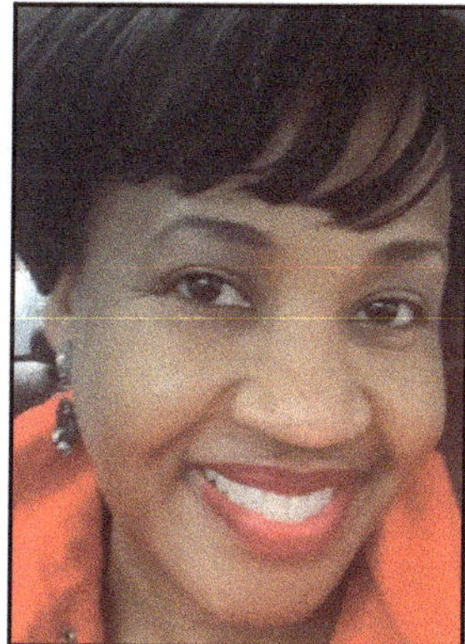 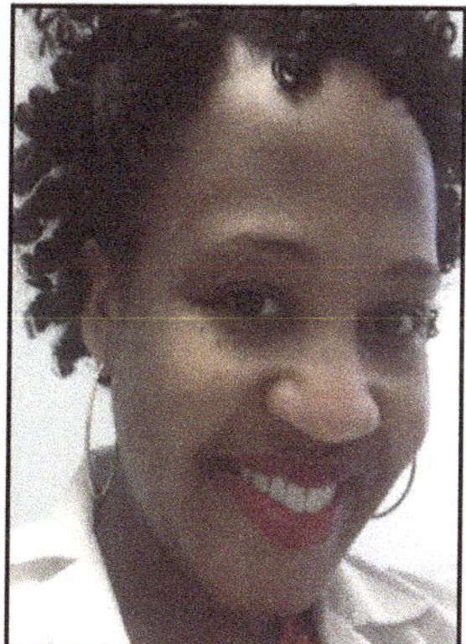

Figure 19A) TWA   **Figure 19B) Silk Press**   **Figure 19C) Perm Rod Set**

NUTRITION AND HAIR

THE ABC'S OF SELF-DIAGNOSIS

There are many benefits to utilizing search engines when you are faced with a health concern. In the age of the internet, we are more informed than ever before, and information that may once have been hidden away in university libraries or medical journals is now available to anyone who has internet access. But it is important to note that the importance of online research does not replace the guidance of your personal healthcare professional. Very often I see individuals go online to obtain recommendations for "hair loss" without taking into account that there are, as you have seen in this book, seventeen different types of hair loss and scalp conditions (or disorders). Then, they go through the ABC's of self-diagnosis.

A is for *Alopecia*, but not Always.

First, many patients give themselves a diagnosis of "alopecia." What I have covered in this book is that there are many different kinds of hair loss or alopecia, which is simply Latin for "the partial or complete absence of hair from areas of the body where it normally grows" by definition. Some hair loss could be due to medication (Telogen Effluvium [TE], see Chapter 2), a fungal infection (Tinea Capitis, see Chapter 7), psoriasis (see Chapter 17), chemotherapy (Anagen Effluvium, see Chapter 9), or a myriad of other causes and conditions. A board-certified dermatologist, preferably one who specializes in hair loss (visit the websites www.carfintl.org or www.docs4hair.com to find one) can diagnose and assist you in navigating the pathway to optimal outcomes. Remember that an early, correct diagnosis yields the most positive results. Self-diagnosis can waste precious time. Time is not only money, time is HAIR FOLLICLES!

B is for *Biotin*, but Biotin is for Breakage.

Ninety to ninety-five percent of my patients come to see me for evaluation of hair loss have already been taking a regimen of biotin before they make their first appointment with me. When individuals realize that they are losing hair, they go online and see that biotin is recommended on blogs and various sources. Almost inevitably, our first appointment is spent on complaints about the ineffectiveness of biotin and sometimes even side effects experienced, including cystic acne and more recently warnings reported by the FDA that high doses of biotin can interfere with hundreds of common lab tests, including some that emergency room doctors use to diagnose a heart attack called troponins to thyroid function tests.[46] Many dietary supplements promoted for hair, skin, and nail benefits can contain biotin levels up to 650 times the recommended daily dose. Researchers at the University

---

46   Biotin (Vitamin B7): Safety Communication - May Interfere with Lab Tests. Downloaded at: www.fda.gov/Safety/MedWatch/SafetyInformation/SafetyAlertsforHumanMedicalProducts/ucm586641.htm

of Minnesota published the results of their study of six healthy adults whom they asked to take 10 mg of biotin (which is a common dose in many hair, skin, and nails vitamin supplements) for one week. About 40% of the blood tests for nine different hormones (including thyroid hormones TSH, Thyroglobulin, T3 and T4), parathyroid hormone, DHEAS, estradiol and ferritin (which, as you many recall from Chapter 2, is often checked in the evaluation of TE) were thrown off after taking the supplements for only one week.[47] A patient might say, "I've been taking Biotin for six months with no improvement." In these cases, Biotin is not the problem; misdiagnosis is. The only time I recommend a trial of Biotin is when I notice a structural problem with the hair that is causing it to break easily. Hair loss, on the other hand, is not a symptom of biotin deficiency. And while some medications can cause biotin levels to decrease, every decrease is not a deficiency. There is no scientific data that proves that individuals without an inherited biotin deficiency benefit from additional supplementation. The majority of data purporting biotin as a solution to hair breakage is based on cases where patients are unable to absorb biotin naturally from food sources. That, I will explain later in this chapter. While certain vitamins are important for the optimal health of your hair, they are more efficiently absorbed from food sources rather than supplements. When these supplements are inevitably ineffective after many months of use, the majority of my biotin-users decide to seek the help of a professional. It is my goal that we change that and the culture around hair loss. My recommended approach is to seek professional help first before wasting precious time, hair follicles, and the unneeded stress, which invariably comes from having uncontrolled hair loss.

---

47 Danni Li, Angela Radulescu, et al. Association of Biotin Ingestion With Performance of Hormone and Nonhormone Assays in Healthy Adults. *AMA*. 2017;318(12):1150–1160.

C is for *Call Your Dermatologist,* but it takes *Courage.*

As I have said multiple times throughout this book, early diagnosis yields the most positive results. So why am I the last step in a person's response to hair loss? There are many reasons, and I will deal with one of the most common reasons: FEAR, an acronym that I love which stands for: False Evidence Appearing Real.

It can be scary to find out what is actually going on when we notice changes, but finding a dermatologist with whom you connect can help to alleviate some of those fears. I know that hair loss is hard to face, but not addressing something does not make it go away. Addressing the problem head-on is the wisest approach and the one that will yield the most successful treatment. If you are still afraid, you should bring someone who cares about you to your appointment. Our loved ones can give us courage and calm our nerves. The number one goal for my patients is to prevent, stabilize, or restore hair loss. Again, an early diagnosis is key to meeting this goal.

Another way to alleviate fear is to learn what happens in an appointment. In an initial appointment, I typically spend time gathering information about your history with hair loss. I depend on my patients to provide me with the clues that will help me to accurately diagnose their condition. To help your dermatologist, you should come prepared with written answers to the following questions:

1. How long have you been experiencing the issue?

2. Are you on a restricted diet of any sort?

3. What medicines are you currently taking or what medicines have you taken in the last few months?

4. Are there any people in your family who are experiencing or have experienced hair loss?

5. Have you tried to treat this condition before? If so, with what treatment?

6. Has a dermatologist or medical professional diagnosed your condition before? If so, did you have a biopsy?

7. Has a medical professional prescribed you medicine to treat this condition? If so, what medicine and what were the results?

Specific answers to these questions will help me avoid duplication of ineffective treatments. Some clients come in and say, "I was given some cream…" The problem is that with hundreds of creams on the market, I might end up prescribing you something similar to what you already had, which produced no results. There is no way to accurately guess which medications were prescribed before. Remember that *you are the expert* on your own history.

WHEN ARE VITAMINS OR SUPPLEMENTS NECESSARY?

There are times when a patient's history will lead me to suspect that vitamin deficiencies may be related to their condition. When this occurs, I order tests to confirm or rule out the deficiencies. Each patient's condition is different, so the following list is by no means a guide to self-diagnosis of vitamin deficiency. Furthermore, ingesting the following list of vitamins does not guarantee that you will not encounter hair loss. But I am a firm believer in doing all that is in your power to protect your hair's health. A healthy diet, along with proper hair care and avoidance of harsh chemicals are within your control.

Regarding these vitamins, it is important whenever possible to get them from food. The vitamins in food are better absorbed by the body than are the vitamin supplements that are sold in tablets or capsules.

Iron

Iron deficiency is ranked as the world's most common nutritional deficiency by the World Health Organization, affecting up to 80 percent of humankind and is a well-known cause of hair loss. What remains unclear is what degree of deficiency may contribute to hair loss.[48] Even in the absence of anemia, diffuse hair loss and other skin symptoms, such as glossitis (inflammation of the tongue), cheilitis (inflammation of the corners of the mouth, and koilonychias (spoon nails), can occur. Iron deficiency can lead to decreased keratin production can lead to thinner anagen hairs. For laboratory tests, sufficient ferritin (the storage form of iron) levels are essential, reflecting how much iron is stored in your tissues. Even though your levels may return in the normal range, I recommend levels of 70 ng/mL for optimal hair health.[49]

---

48 Guo EL and Katta R. Diet and hair loss: effects of nutrient deficiency and supplement use. Dermatol Pract Concept. 2017 Jan; 7(1): 1–10.

49 Lenzy, YM. Dr. Lenzy's Hair Diet: 11 Tips to Achieve Your Best Hair Ever! Available at: http://www.lenzyderm.com/hair-diet-e-book/

In premenopausal women, iron deficiency is often due to menorrhagia or pregnancy, whereas, especially in older patients, gastrointestinal bleeding should be excluded.

The recommended ferritin levels and their significance for hair loss are still an object of scientific discussion, with several studies coming to different conclusions.[50]

Many authors consider a ferritin level of at least 40 mg/L as adequate in their female patients; others only require 10 mg/L, and some require 70 mg/L. To correct iron deficiency, ferrous fumarate, ferrous lactate, ferrous gluconate, or ferrous sulfate are different forms of iron that can be taken for several weeks in two to three daily doses, because absorption is lower in high doses. The latter two formulations may be better tolerated. For the treatment of low iron deficiency anemia, the Centers for Disease Control and Prevention recommends 50 to 60 mg of oral elemental iron twice daily for three months, which corresponds to 325 mg of ferrous sulfate twice a day.

Foods that are rich in iron include: red meat, pork, poultry, seafood, beans, dark, green-leafy vegetables (such as spinach and kale), dried fruit (such as raisins and dates), iron-fortified grains, and peas. Additionally, foods that are rich in vitamin C can also help the body to absorb more iron. These foods include: broccoli, grapefruit, kiwi, leafy greens, melons, oranges, peppers, strawberries, tangerines, and tomatoes, just to name a few.[51] One cup of guava has 377 mg of vitamin C (more than 4 times the minimum

---

50 Guo EL and Katta R. Diet and hair loss: effects of nutrient deficiency and supplement use. <u>Dermatol Pract Concept</u>. 2017 Jan; 7(1): 1–10.

51 http://www.mayoclinic.org/diseases-conditions/iron-deficiency-anemia/basics/prevention/con-20019327

daily recommended amount) and [52]yellow peppers have nearly 5.5 times more vitamin c than oranges (341 mg vs 63 mg).[53]

Zinc

Zinc is an essential mineral required by hundreds of enzymes and transcription factors required for protein synthesis and cell division. The required daily zinc uptake of 8 to 10 mg per day is usually supplied through a normal diet, but deficiencies are still common in developing countries. Zinc deficiency can lead to Telogen Effluvium, thin white, brittle hair, as well as nail dystrophy. Acquired zinc deficiency occurs in elderly persons, in persons with alcoholism, anorexia nervosa, nephropathy, and pancreatitis. In addition, zinc deficiency can occur after prolonged breast feeding without supplementation, following gastrointestinal bypass surgery, from consuming cereals containing phytate (which binds phytate and prevents absorption), having an excessive intake of iron, and after taking medications that chelate zinc, such as diuretics, valproic acid, penicillamine angiotensin-converting enzyme inhibitors.[54]

During treatment, zinc levels should be monitored because overdose can lead to copper or calcium deficiency, drowsiness, and headache. The daily reference intake for men and pregnant women is 11 mg and for women is 8 mg. In deficiency, the recommended dose for adults is 25 to 50 mg of elemental zinc and 0.5 to 1 mg/kg for children. Although traditionally used in unspecific hair treatments, an effect of zinc supplementation on hair growth

52   Guo EL and Katta R. Diet and hair loss: effects of nutrient deficiency and supplement use. Dermatol Pract Concept. 2017 Jan; 7(1): 1–10.

53   Lenzy, YM. Dr. Lenzy's Hair Diet: 11 Tips to Achieve Your Best Hair Ever! Available at: http://www.lenzyderm.com/hair-diet-e-book/

in patients with normal serum zinc levels has not been sufficiently proven.

Foods that are rich in zinc include: seafood (such as oysters, shrimp and mussels), red meat, poultry, dairy products, including yogurt and cheese, nuts and beans, cashews and almonds, and zinc-fortified cereals.[54] A study was conducted with 30 health controls and 312 patients who were diagnosed with alopecia areata (AA), male pattern hair loss, female pattern hair loss, and telogen effluvium (TE). In all of the hair loss patients, the mean serum zinc was 84.33, significantly lower than the control group (97.94±21.05 ng/dl), which was statistically significant). The analysis of each group showed that all groups of hair loss had statistically lower zinc concentration. However, the ratio of the patients with serum zinc concentration lower than 70 ng/dl was significantly high in only the AA group (odds ratio, OR 4.02) and the TE group (OR 1.12). Conclusion: The data led to the hypothesis of zinc metabolism disturbances playing a key role in hair loss, especially AA and TE.[55]

Vitamin A

Although vitamin A deficiency is not an established cause of hair loss, an excessive intake can lead to general hair loss and dry skin. The recommended maximum daily intake is 10,000 IU. For this reason, I am not a fan of "hair vitamins" that contain >5,000 IU or 163% the recommended daily allowance.[56]

---

54   http://healthyeating.sfgate.com/foods-rich-zinc-vitamin-b-8584.html

55   Min SK, Chul WK, Sang SK. Analysis of Serum Zinc and Copper Concentrations in Hair Loss. *Ann Dermatol.* 2013 Nov; 25(4):405–409.

56   Lenzy, YM. Dr. Lenzy's Hair Diet: 11 Tips to Achieve Your Best Hair Ever! Available at: http://www.lenzyderm.com/hair-diet-e-book/

Vitamin D

Data from animal studies suggest that vitamin D plays a role in hair follicle cycling. Studies have shown an increase in vitamin D receptor expression in the outer root sheath of the hair follicle during the growing phase of the hair cycle.[57] In a study of AA, levels of vitamin D were lower in AA patients when compared to healthy controls with a significant correlation between more severe AA and lower vitamin D levels.[58]

Obtaining a vitamin D3 level in patients with TE can be helpful. There are many sources of vitamin D, including: sunlight, fatty fish, canned tuna, certain mushrooms, fortified milk, egg yolks, beef liver, and fortified cereal.[59] The reference daily intake for adults is 5 to 10 µg (1 µg calciferol = 40 IU vitamin D).

Vitamin H (Biotin)

Biotin deficiency is rare because it is also produced by intestinal bacteria. It has been seen in congenital or acquired biotinidase or carboxylase deficiency, in tube feedings, in individuals with impaired gastrointestinal flora caused by antibiotics, and after excessive ingestion of raw white eggs due to binding by a protein found in egg whites called avidin. Symptoms include structural changes of the hair and nails, perioral dermatitis, conjunctivitis, and infections. Alopecia is not a typical symptom of biotin deficiency but trichorrhexis nodosa and other structural anomalies can

---

57   Guo EL and Katta R. Diet and hair loss: effects of nutrient deficiency and supplement use. Dermatol Pract Concept. 2017 Jan; 7(1):1–10.

58   Bhat YJ, Latif I, et al. Vitamin D Level in Alopecia Areata. *Indian J Dermatol.* 2017 Jul-Aug; 62(4):407–410.

59   http://www.health.com/health/gallery/0,,20504538,00.html

occur. The reference daily intake for adults is 30 mg. Antiepileptic drugs can reduce biotin levels. In those cases, a prophylactic supplementation can therefore be recommended.

It has not been sufficiently shown that additional supplementation of biotin in patients with normal blood levels can improve hair loss, although an effect on hair and nail structure is possible.

FROM THE BLOGS: RICE WATER FOR HAIR HEALTH

Over the past year, there has been a surge in the number of internet searches for "rice water for hair" as well as inquires in my inbox that I wanted to include a word on it here. In terms of internet beauty blogs, rice water is listed as having several hair benefits, including "adding shine to your hair and helping to keep it strong and healthy"[60] via it containing "inositol, a carbohydrate that helps strengthen elasticity and reduce surface friction."[14] The same blog states that "rice water is full of vitamins and minerals that are wonderful for both hair and skin, something women in Asian cultures have known for centuries." Because of this, I searched for evidenced-based articles published to corroborate these claims since it has been reportedly practices for centuries in Asian beauty culture. A search of "rice water and hair" in Pub Med (the National Library of Medicine's repository of peer-reviewed research) yielded no results, but I found an abstract published in the *International Journal of Cosmetic Chemistry*, which "examined the Yu-Su-Ru (rinse water obtained from the washing of rice) hair care practice in the Heian Period, and examined its effects on hair. They

---

60   One Good Thing By Jillee Blog. "The Beauty Benefits of Rice Water." Downloaded April 22, 2018, at https://www.onegoodthingbyjillee.com/2015/04/the-beauty-benefits-of-rice-water.html

published that "Yu-Su-Ru exhibited hair care effects, such as reducing surface friction and increasing hair elasticity. However, when hair was treated with Yu-Su-Ru alone, flaking was observed on the hair surface, and the direct application of Yu-Su-Ru was considered difficult. Thus, Yu-Su-Ru extracts, which are highly effective in hair care and did not cause flaking were examined. These results showed that Yu-Su-Ru extracts had multiple functions for hair care at the same time. Thus, the new application of Yu-Su-Ru for hair care was discovered."[61] The abstract failed to detail the specifics of what the "multiple functions" were. Regarding the claims of rice water aiding in hair loss, I found no evidence base to this claim. Given that the practice appears to be safe, I have no recommendation against it but would prefer to see this examined in a well-designed study with one group using rice water compared with another group using no rice water to better isolate the effect on various forms of hair loss.

A NOTE ON SPECIAL (OR FAD?) DIETS ON HAIR AND HEALTH

Blood Type Diet

Over the past decade, diets that are based on the ABO blood type system have been promoted and claim to improve health and decrease risk of disease. The ABO blood typing is typically correlated with blood transfusions because the ABO blood product incompatibility can potentially prove fatal. More recently, the use of genome-wide association studies (GWAS) have supported a number

---

61 Inamasu S, Ikuyama et al. The Effect of Rinse Water Obtained from the Washing of Rice (YU-SU-RU) as a Hair Treatment. *Journal of Cosmetic Chemists Volume.* 2010;44(1):29–33.

of associations between ABO blood type and certain diseases, including pancreatic cancer, venous blood clots, and cardiovascular disease. Therefore, it appears *possible* that ABO blood group plays a role in determining an individual's susceptibility to certain diseases. This established association between blood types and disease has been the basis for a range of diets. Of the many author's blood type diets[62,63], D'Adamo is arguably the most popular with his initial book, published in 1996, with >7 million copies in print.[64] D'Adamo claims that each ABO blood type processes food differently, and adherence to a diet specific to an individual's ABO blood type could improve health, well-being and energy, and reduce risk of developing certain diseases such as cancer and cardiovascular disease. D'Adamo's diets are "based on a theory that each blood type contains the genetic message of the diets and behaviors of our ancestors and these traits still impact us today."[65] Considering the substantial reach of the blood type diets, it is pertinent to be able to substantiate the health claims of blood type diets so that inquiries to physicians and dieticians can be adequately addressed.

Using my method of evaluating the strength of health recommendations, I performed a PubMed search for "blood type diet" and found the only systematic review examining the scientific evidence to support the effectiveness of blood type diets published in the *American Journal of Clinical Nutrition*. In the systematic

---

62 Christiano J. Joseph Christiano's blood type diet O: a custom eating plan for losing weight, fighting disease, and staying healthy for people with type O blood. Lake Mary, FL: Siloam, 2010.

63 Wilson M. Blood type diet: O, A, B, AB eating the best recipes to make you healthy: lose weight, be healthier and stronger with the blood type diet guide. Kindle ed. CreateSpace Independent Publishing Platform, 2011.

64 D'Adamo PJ. Eat right 4 your blood type. New York, NY: GP Putnam Son's, 1996.

65 Cusack L, De Buck E, et al. Blood type diets lack supporting evidence: a systematic review. *Am J Clin Nutr*. 2013;98:99–104.

review, published studies that presented data related to blood type diets were identified and critically appraised using the Grading of Recommendations, Assessment, Development, and Evaluation (GRADE) approach. The systemic search was performed to answer the question: In humans grouped according to blood type, does adherence to a specific diet improve health and/or decrease risk of disease compared with nonadherence to diet? Out of 1415 screened references, 16 articles were identified with only one considered eligible according to the selection criteria. The identified article studied the variation the variation between LDL-cholesterol responses of different MNS blood types to a low-fat diet. No studies that showed the health effects of ABO blood type diets were identified. Therefore, the systematic review concluded that NO EVIDENCE currently exists to validate the purported health benefits of blood type diets. To validate these claims, studies are required that compare the health outcomes between participants adhering to a particular blood type diet (experimental group) and participants continuing a standard diet (control group) within a particular blood group.

INTERMITTENT FASTING

Overweight and obesity (classified as a Body Mass Index [BMI] of greater than 25 and 30, respectively) are global public health concerns with over 1.9 billion adults worldwide being overweight and 600 million obese. A raised BMI in adulthood is associated with an increased risk of developing a number of chronic diseases, which include diabetes, cardiovascular disease, muscular skeletal disorders like osteoarthritis, and some cancers. Effective weight management is challenging and while a plethora of available weight loss programs exist, not all are completely evaluated and compared, and many weight loss attempts result in weight regain and poor long-term results.[66] It is therefore important to review the effectiveness of new approaches to support and evidenced-based approach to weight management. Intermittent energy restriction encompasses dietary approaches, including intermittent fasting (IF), alternate day fasting, or fasting for two days per week. These approaches involve interspersing normal daily caloric intake with a short period of severe calorie restriction/fasting. IF regimens have gained considerable popularity in recent years, as some people find these diets easier to follow than traditional calorie restriction approaches. A recent systematic review and meta-analysis (which involves polling the results of multiple studies together) was conducted to examine the effectiveness or IF in the treatment of overweight and obesity in adults when compared to usual care treatment or no treatment.[67] Six studies were included in the review ranging in duration from three to 12 months, with four studies including continuous energy restriction as a comparator intervention and two studies including a no treatment control group. Meta-analyses showed that intermittent restriction was statistically significantly more effective than no treatment for weight loss (loss of 9.1 lbs., p<0.001). The pooled estimate for studies that investigated the effect of intermittent energy restriction in comparison to continuous energy restriction revealed no significant difference in weight loss (loss of 2.3 lbs., *p*=0.156). Therefore, the systematic review concluded that intermittent energy restriction may be an effective strategy

---

66   Jane L, et al. Intermittent fasting interventions for the treatment of overweight and obesity in adults aged 18 years and over: a systematic review protocol. *JBI Database System Rev Implement Rep.* 2015 Oct;13(10):60–68.

67   Harris L, et al. Intermittent fasting interventions for treatment of overweight and obesity in adults: a systematic review and meta-analysis. *JBI Database System Rev Implement Rep.* 2018 Feb;16(2):507–547.

for the treatment of overweight and obesity and was comparable to continuous energy restriction for short-term weight loss in overweight and obese adults, with the caveat being to interpret the results cautiously given the small number of studies.

SUMMARY: THE ABC'S OF EFFECTIVE TREATMENT

In sharing the ABC's of self-diagnosis, I have described the missteps that can occur in response to hair loss, the truth about biotin, the importance of knowing your medical history, and a summary of my research on the correlation between vitamin deficiency (or excess) and certain types of hair loss. Now, I will share the ABC's of effective treatment.

A is for Awareness: When you first begin to notice excessive shedding, small bald patches, breakage, or thinning hair, you should write down what you notice. Be specific. Although a medical professional can best diagnose your condition, you are the expert on your own symptoms. Be aware. The Cicatricial Alopecia Research Foundation (CARF) is a great resource to improve patient awareness about the cicatricial or scarring alopecias (www.carfintl.org). The National Alopecia Areata Foundation is a great resource for individuals diagnosed with Alopecia Areata (www.naaf.org).

B is for Breathe: Sometimes awareness of symptoms can send us hunting down the rabbit hole of internet research. But panic only delays progress, as it can sidetrack us with unhelpful home remedies. Remember to breathe. Keep calm and...

C is for Call your Dermatologist: I cannot emphasize enough the importance of early diagnosis. I cannot offer a guarantee of successful treatment if "success" means the complete reversal of a condition. But if "success" is defined as the journey to identifying, then treating, a specific condition, then I will say that a successful treatment depends on your connection to a medical professional who can: 1) calm some of your fears, 2) help to guide your research (let's face it: we're not giving up our search engines anytime soon), 3) take the steps necessary to accurately diagnose your condition, and 4) provide you with options for treatment or prevention.

If you or someone you know is just beginning to notice hair loss, I hope that this book has given you the information and guidance necessary for you to begin the healing journey. The Cicatricial Alopecia Research Foundation (CARF), a patient-centered organization that provides information, support, and funding for research on the scarring alopecias, has compiled a listing of licensed dermatologists who specialize in hair loss and hair care. Their website, www.carfintl.org, has free educational brochures that include helpful images of various conditions. CARF was started by a patient and her dermatologist, in whom she found a caring partner in the journey toward healing. I wish the same for you or your loved one. Docs4hair.com is another resource to located Dermatologists who specialize in hair loss as well as hair stylists and trichologists who partner with dermatologists to provide a teach-based approach to providing excellent hair and scalp treatment.

LET'S KEEP THE CONVERSATION GOING!

Please join our Facebook Community, "Healthy Hair, Skin, and Bodies with Dr. Lenzy" and www.exerciseandhair.com. I update the page with new information about prevention and treatment of hair loss and fitness tips and tricks. You can submit questions to me that I will answer for the group's benefit. Most important, you will find a community of people who may be going through a similar journey.

For those of you who are licensed cosmetologists or planning to pursue a career in hair loss or trichology, I have developed a 12-week online training program to help you up-level your knowledge to better serve your clients dealing with hair loss on my website www.gettingtotherootbook.com. Come learn how you can best serve clients who are experiencing breakage, damage, or loss. Beauty professionals are on the front line to help clients achieve an earlier diagnosis, which will ultimately provide better treatment outcomes!

PRAISE FOR THE BOOK

Many students completing my classes went on to great things. Dr. Yolanda Lenzy was a student that went above and beyond: first, by convincing the school system to allow her to pursue both an academic path and a vocational education path, which is unheard of even to this dayj; second, by excelling in the cosmetology program; and third, embracing the Vocational Industrial Clubs of America (VICA) now known as

SkillUSA. She was elected to a Maryland State Office (Historian) and followed that by being elected to the office of National Vice President. Dr. Lenzy set a path for herself and did what it takes to reach the end goal. We have had many conversations over the years, and I marvel at her passion to help others with dedication and drive to keep digging until she has answers to solve each situation. *Getting to the Root* is wonderful tool for anyone who needs information on hair loss conditions. Keep all of your passions going!

Melanie Stancliff
Cosmetology Instructor
Laurel Senior High School
Laurel, MD

Dr. Lenzy has created a bridge from patient to caregiver. In *Getting to the Root*, she successfully channels her expertise and experience into a must-have primer for anyone suffering with hair loss. A great resource.

Lynne J. Goldberg, M.D.
Professor of Dermatology at Boston University
and Director of the Hair Clinic
Boston Medical Center
Boston, MA

We discovered Dr. Yolanda during the early days of her Facebook show: #LunchNLearn with Dr. Yolanda. The first broadcast I viewed was her sharing her journey into medicine. As I watched with tears freely falling down my face, I didn't just hear her story, I felt it! I immediately shared it with my daughter, my friends, and their daughters. Of course, there was no question that we would schedule a virtual consultation immediately. My daughter needed some guidance on combating a skin condition Dr. Lenzy diagnosed as seborrheic dermatitis. She took the time to not only provide a clear treatment plan but the most impactful take-away was how she poured into my daughter. It wasn't the cookie-cutter, aloof physician-to-patient interaction that we were accustomed to. She genuinely took the time to hear my daughter's educational goals that were followed by heartfelt words of encouragement. Based on the incomparable content provided on her show, #LunchNLearn, and the effective, unforgettable virtual consultation received, we believe that *Getting to the Root* will impact generations. We are deeply appreciative that the Lord gifted the world with Dr. Yolanda and we are blessed to be beneficiaries!

Monetta Fields
Laurel, MD

Dr. Yolanda Lenzy is not just a phenomenal doctor but a beautiful person as well. I will never forget my first interaction with her, which was a virtual consultation. After she completed the examination, we began to engage in conversation that was both organic and true. She asked me about my college life and what my goals, aspirations, and dreams were. It was obvious how much she cared about people and wanted to help me in any way possible. Dr. Lenzy is a light and an inspiration. I am so grateful to have met her.

Kyla Fields
Virtual Consultation Patient
Laurel, MD

I met Dr. Lenzy virtually around 2015 and have been following her via social media on her show, #LunchNLearn ever since. I suffered from a scalp condition for about a year before contacting her. I was embarrassed for months and decreased my trips to the hair salon because of it. My hair stylist suggested a product line that would work initially but the scalp plague would return to no avail. While I do still have flare ups, the diagnosis and treatment Dr. Lenzy provided has been working when I use it consistently. She has changed my life personally and professionally serving as her on-air live stream transcription assistant or during the best in evidence-based medicine shared on social media during #LunchNLearn.

Getting to the Root: A Dermatologist's & Cosmetologist's Guide to Understanding HAIR is a comprehensive conversational encyclopedia of how hair conditions affect us all on a daily basis. This guide begins in Dr. Lenzy's own family and leads us through evidence-based medicine, patient encounters, and brings us all into hope and healing regarding our hair and overall health. Everyone from doctors to daughters should share this extensive, useful guide since we need this as a community, and you'll learn and lead by passing this on to someone else!"

De'Nita Moss
Virtual Consultation Patient
#LunchNLearn Scribe @TrinityScribes
New Jersey